# RUN YOUR BEST MARATHON

# RUN YOUR BEST MARATHON

## Your trusted guide to training and racing better

### Sam Murphy

BLOOMSBURY SPORT

LONDON · OXFORD · NEW YORK · NEW DELHI · SYDNEY

BLOOMSBURY SPORT
Bloomsbury Publishing Plc
50 Bedford Square, London, WC1B 3DP, UK
29 Earlsfort Terrace, Dublin 2, Ireland

BLOOMSBURY, BLOOMSBURY SPORT and the Diana logo are trademarks of
Bloomsbury Publishing Plc

First published in Great Britain 2022

A catalogue record for this book is available from the British Library

Library of Congress Cataloguing-in-Publication data has been applied for

ISBN: 978-1-4729-8952-9; eBook: 978-1-4729-8953-6

2 4 6 8 10 9 7 5 3 1

Typeset in Spectral Light by Deanta Global Publishing Services, Chennai, India
Printed and bound in Great Britain by CPI Group (UK) Ltd, Croydon, CR0 4YY

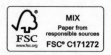

To find out more about our authors and books visit www.bloomsbury.com and
sign up for our newsletters

# CONTENTS

# INTRODUCTION

This is a book for runners. You might not be a marathon runner yet, but you have enough miles under your belt to understand that there's more to running than putting one foot in front of the other. You've seen how it gives you a chance to find out what you're made of, to discover untapped resourcefulness and determination, to experience the thrill of overcoming obstacles and accomplishing goals. Whether you run alone or with others, you've probably felt that sense of being part of something bigger – the ever-growing community who find pleasure, challenge, meaning and fun in this simple act.

Runners of all persuasions get this. But there *is* something magical about the marathon. I was 22 when I ran my first one – not London, but Luton. My mum drove me to the race and we passed a sign on the motorway that read 'Luton 26'. Those 26 miles (42km) seemed to take an age to cover in the car, filling me with fear and doubt about my abilities to *run* so far. But I did. And like many runners who believe we are only ever going to do 'one', I found myself in the hours, days and weeks afterwards wondering: should I have done X in training? Would Y have made me run quicker? If I'd done Z, maybe I wouldn't have hit the wall... Before I knew it, I was signing up to another 26.2, and another.

You might have experienced something the same. Or perhaps you've not yet crossed a marathon finish line. Either way, this book is for you. I'm well aware that there is already a wealth of information on running marathons out there, from websites and apps to podcasts, magazines and other books. But I wrote this particular book with some specific aims in mind.

First, to guide you through the latest evidence-based information and advice on every aspect of marathon training and racing – without blinding you with science. Second, to present this information and advice in a way that allows you to make the best decisions about which bits are most relevant and important to *you*. For example, if your goal is to just complete the distance with a big grin on your face, the training priorities may be different than for someone who has a set goal time in mind. If you're one giant niggle in running shoes, you might take a different approach to someone who rarely gets injured.

Much of the information derived from sports science research and coaching comes from those working with elite performers. Simply extrapolating those findings doesn't always work, because those athletes' natural talent – and the fact that they are pursuing running as a career – sets them apart. One study found that elite Kenyan runners train 10–14 times a week. I don't, and I'm guessing you don't either.

I'll give you an example of how extrapolation from the elites can fall down. It's often advised that the long run should comprise 20–25 per cent of weekly mileage. That's fine, if you're running 80 miles (129km) a week – but what if you're running 30 miles (48km)? How will you get to the higher reaches of those long runs without breaking the 'rule'? You need to consider the science, but within the context of the *real* world of the amateur runner with limitations and commitments – practical, physical, social, mental – other than running to fit into our lives.

My marathon-training programmes are not based on set time goals, because every runner embarking on them is unique. Instead, they are based on training volume – you might be limited in terms of how much you can do by time availability, inclination, energy levels or injury vulnerability, so there are different commitment levels (from three days a week to five or six days a week) with options for first-timers and those aiming to improve on an existing time within each level. But you may decide, having read this book, that you want to devise your own training plan – and you will be equipped with the tools to do so.

One of the biggest mistakes I find people make with marathon training is leaving themselves out of the equation. They decide, for example, that they'd like to run a sub-3 hrs 30 mins marathon and find a 'Run sub-3 hrs 30 mins plan' to follow. But this plan 'knows' nothing about the runner: their previous experience, their fitness level, age, injury propensity, training availability, mental attitude, lifestyle – all of which influence what is achievable. Not only is it impossible for the plan to guide everyone who follows it to a 3 hrs 29 mins finish, it may also represent way too much training for one runner, not enough for another and simply the wrong emphasis for yet another.

It's one thing to know a lot about the marathon – quite another to know a lot about yourself as a runner. Fitting the two together is what makes coaching both an art and a science – and is the challenge that has kept me fascinated for the last two decades.

While you're in marathon training – a fact you'll already be aware of if you've run marathons before (as will your partner/family!) – it will occupy a lot of your time and thoughts. And rightly so, because what you do outside of those few hours a week when you are running greatly affects how well your body 'absorbs' the training you undertake. That's why I cover sleep, nutrition and stress within the pages of this book.

While training errors (too little, too much or the wrong kind) are the main reason people underperform in the marathon, race-day mistakes are a close second. Did you know that running just 2 per cent too fast over the first 6 miles (10km) of a marathon is likely to cause you to slow over the final miles? Or that the best time to take your first energy gel is before you've even started running? There are physical quandaries to consider, too, like how to race on a hot day, how to get in enough fuel and fluid without upsetting your guts, as well as mental challenges – start-line nerves, loss of focus, negative self-talk – to overcome. I've included a whole section on race-day preparation and race execution to help get you from the start line to the finish line to the best of your ability.

So many things need to come together to create the perfect race. But rather than being daunted or put off by this, the way to see it is that there is always something you can address, tweak or improve on, be it your training strategy, your race plan, your psychological skills, your recovery ritual, your energy intake. And that means there's always another reason to get back on that start line. I hope to see you there.

# ON TRAINING

# 1
# FROM RUNNER TO MARATHONER

## Why the marathon is more than just another race

One of the things I realise anew each time I run a marathon is that 26.2 miles – or 42.2km – is a *long* way. Whether you are tackling the distance for the first time or the umpteenth, the challenge of running that far – at pace – does not diminish. The marathon asks a lot from your body, taking you into realms untouched by shorter-distance events. You could argue that ultramarathons do the same, but here the focus tends to shift from 'How *fast* can I finish?' to '*Can* I finish?', which subtly changes the demands of the race.

The marathon requires not just the physiological and musculoskeletal endurance to 'keep going', but also the stamina to do so at your goal pace, which necessitates efficient fuel utilisation (I'm not talking about how many gels you can stomach but about how well your body uses fat and carbohydrates to produce energy).

It's not just your body that gets pushed to its limits. In the early miles, you'll need to draw on discipline and self-control to manage your pace and not get carried away; later in the race, you'll face the struggle to stay focused and maintain a positive mindset, and in the last miles – when your body is clamouring for you to stop or slow down – you'll need to summon up the last vestiges of your mental strength to ignore it and push on to the finish. Some of these challenges apply to any race – a 10K or half-marathon, for example. But in other respects, the marathon is unique.

The sheer distance – or length of time – that you're on your feet for is the main factor that separates the marathon from other races. In the process of running 26.2 miles (42.2km), you'll take over 40,000 strides, with a force of two to three times your bodyweight being exerted on each landing. If you weigh 70kg (11 stone), that's a force equivalent to around 7 million kg (7000 tonnes) going through your joints, putting a lot of strain on the musculoskeletal system (bones, muscles and connective tissue, like cartilage and tendons). Then there's the need to take fuel and fluid on board (you'll burn somewhere in the region of 3000 calories over the course of the race, emptying your body's stores of carbohydrate and sweating out 4 litres/7 pints of fluid) – and the prospect of dealing with setbacks such as muscle cramps, a rebellious stomach, chafing and blisters.

The issue of fuel utilisation, which I mentioned above (in fact, you'll probably get sick of me mentioning it!), is another marathon-specific challenge. Runners are unlikely to 'run out' of fuel in ultramarathons because the pace they are running at (relative to their marathon pace) is slower. The same is true in shorter races, because they reach the finish before the body's stores are depleted. (I'll explain more about this later in this chapter.)

For all these reasons, I don't view the marathon as 'just another race'. Not if you want to run it well, anyway. (And by 'well', I don't necessarily mean fast – I mean getting out of it what you hoped to.) To master the marathon, you need an understanding of what it requires from your body and what type of training will enable your body to adapt to those demands. You also need to know where you stand – what your starting point is – so you can plan appropriate training and allow enough time for those adaptations to take place. Let's start by looking at the key attributes of a good marathon runner.

# What makes a marathoner?

- ☑ Good cardiovascular (aerobic) fitness – to bring as much oxygen as possible into the body and deliver it to the working muscles.
- ☑ Good running economy – to use that oxygen efficiently.
- ☑ A high lactate threshold – to maintain a high proportion of maximal aerobic capacity ($VO_2$ max) for the duration of the marathon.
- ☑ Efficient fuel utilisation – to utilise a higher proportion of fat to produce energy at goal pace and conserve precious glycogen stores.
- ☑ Fatigue-resistant muscles – a higher proportion of fatigue-resistant 'slow-twitch' muscle fibres and a larger 'workforce' of recruitable muscle fibres allow muscles to contract repeatedly over a prolonged period without failing.
- ☑ A robust musculoskeletal system – to prevent injury.
- ☑ The right mindset and psychological skills for training and racing.
- ☑ The capacity to recover well and quickly from training.

Over the next few pages, we're going to delve further into why these attributes matter for marathon running.

## Cardiovascular fitness

Ninety-nine per cent of the energy required to run a marathon is produced aerobically ('with oxygen'). And cardiovascular or aerobic fitness is all about the ability of the heart, lungs and blood to bring that oxygen into the body and transport it to the working muscles during exercise. There are a number of ways in which running (or any aerobic activity) improves the efficiency with which your body can do this (see 'How training affects your cardiovascular system' on the following page).

# HOW TRAINING AFFECTS YOUR CARDIOVASCULAR SYSTEM

A stronger heart can pump out more blood per beat (stroke volume) and per minute (cardiac output) while a training-induced increase in blood volume (yes, you can actually make more blood!) means more red blood cells – the all-important oxygen-carrying molecules. When the oxygen-rich blood arrives at the muscles, the capillaries surrounding each muscle allow the oxygen to pass through their flimsy walls (and allow waste products to pass out). The more capillaries you have, the more oxygen can diffuse into the muscles – an increase in the capillary network is one of the important effects of endurance training. One study found 33 per cent higher capillarisation in endurance athletes compared to non-active people.

There are two things that determine how much of the delivered oxygen gets *used* within the muscle to produce the energy required for running. The abundance of aerobic enzymes (essentially, enzymes are substances that facilitate chemical reactions) and the number, size and efficiency of the mitochondria, which are tiny structures that reside in every cell and specialise in aerobic energy production. All types and intensities of exercise boost mitochondrial function, but studies suggest that an intensity equal to or above the lactate threshold is most effective, particularly in older athletes.

You've probably heard the term '$VO_2$ max' (maximal aerobic capacity). This is a measure of how much oxygen can be utilised during *maximal* aerobic exercise, and is expressed as ml of oxygen, per kg of bodyweight, per minute. $VO_2$ max is often wheeled out as the gold standard measure of endurance, and while it's true that you won't find a world-class marathoner with a really poor $VO_2$ max (the average sedentary male may have a $VO_2$ max of 35–45ml/kg/min while a well-trained marathon runner may be closer to 65ml/kg/min and an elite runner

80ml/kg/min) it is important to stress that $VO_2$ max and endurance performance are not the same thing. Research has demonstrated that $VO_2$ max can improve without an uptick in endurance performance – and vice versa.

When scientists have tried to predict marathon performance from $VO_2$ max scores, they've failed miserably. This is because we don't run 26.2 miles at maximal aerobic capacity – it's simply not possible to sustain $VO_2$ max pace for that long. Even over 5K, an elite runner will typically be operating slightly below their $VO_2$ max (around 98 per cent of it). What matters is the *proportion* of maximal capacity that can be sustained in a marathon – and this is where two other physiological variables come into play.

## Running economy

The first is 'running economy'. This is all about efficient use of all that oxygen you've brought into your body. If we take two runners with an equally high $VO_2$ max and get them to run at the same speed, the more economical runner will 'spend' less oxygen doing so, meaning their performance will be less limited by the availability of oxygen in the working muscles. Another way of looking at it is that if you improve your economy, you will either be able to run at any given pace (say, 8-minute-miling) using *less* oxygen than you did before, or run at a *faster* pace using the same amount that you used to need to hit 8-minute-miling. Think of it as your 'miles per gallon' rate. One study found that running economy explained 65 per cent of the variation in endurance performance.

So how do you become more economical? Research suggests that running itself – both how much you run and the length of time you have been a regular runner – plays a role in enhancing economy, probably because it improves the muscles' oxidative capacity (their ability to take in oxygen) and neuromuscular efficiency (the communication between the brain and the muscles). Efficient running economy, built up over decades of training, is one of the reasons many lifelong runners continue to perform well as the years advance. If you're newer to running, it'll take time to reach your peak.

However, there are two stones not to leave unturned if you want to optimise your running economy. Studies show that strength training can have a significant effect, particularly plyometric training, which we look at in Chapter 11. Good running form (covered in Chapter 10) is another important factor. When we tire, running form tends to deteriorate (just watch runners at mile 20 of a marathon, compared to mile 2!), which dents running economy. Working on developing a more biomechanically efficient stride helps direct all your precious energy into propelling you forwards, not rocking side to side or bouncing up and down. It also helps minimise the risk of injuries. Bonus!

## Lactate threshold

The second aspect of cardiovascular fitness that is key to a marathon runner is the oft-discussed 'lactate threshold' (LT). Contrary to popular belief, there is nothing inherently evil about lactate. It is a by-product of the metabolism of carbohydrates, which is recycled to be used as a source of fuel. At leisurely running speeds, not much lactate is produced and it can easily be cleared from the muscles. But as pace increases, so does lactate production, until it reaches the point at which it is being produced more quickly than it can be cleared, leading to an accumulation within the muscle. This makes the environment within the muscle very acidic, hampering muscle contraction and forcing you to slow down.

An average runner might hit lactate threshold at around 75 per cent of their $VO_2$ max, while a more accomplished athlete might be closer to 85 or even 90 per cent. The higher the threshold, the more of their maximal aerobic capacity a runner can make use of, hence, the faster the pace they can sustain. Research suggests that the lactate threshold is the most important determinant of performance in races lasting 30 minutes or more. So if you can nudge the lactate threshold upwards through the right kind of training, you have a good chance of improving marathon performance. In Chapter 2, we look at what 'the right kind of training' involves, as well as how to figure out your own LT.

## Efficient fuel utilisation

Running a marathon requires a lot of energy. To understand how your body produces energy, you need to get familiar with a substance called adenosine triphosphate (ATP). ATP is the molecule involved in converting food into usable energy. However, the amount of ATP stored in your muscles is barely enough to run 26m, let alone 26 miles! Elite marathon coach Renato Canova estimates that the ATP required to run a marathon would weigh a whopping 50kg (110lb). So, instead of carrying ATP, your body needs to constantly resynthesise it. A good way to view ATP is like a bank card – it provides access to cash (energy) without weighing you down.

To access your energy account, you need a steady supply of oxygen and fuel – either glucose (from carbohydrate) or fatty acids (from fat). At low exercise intensities, fat is the preferred fuel source. No problems there – even the leanest runners have a generous supply. But when you're running at anything other than the easiest of efforts, your body relies more on the breakdown of carbohydrate, which can be metabolised more rapidly. And here we hit another storage problem: there is only enough carbohydrate (stored as glycogen in the muscles and liver) to run at a sustained effort for around 90–120 minutes. Once these stores have been depleted, we are forced to rely on the more long-winded process of breaking down fat, which slows us down.

If, however, you can a) improve glycogen storage and b) get better at using fat as a fuel source at marathon pace, you are far less likely to run into energy problems. Research shows that a high volume of training and long runs can help to increase glycogen storage – well-trained runners can store as much as 40 per cent more glycogen than non-exercisers. Moderate-paced runs, sometimes called 'aerobic threshold runs' (think 'a little bit faster than easy') and long runs with bouts of marathon-pace running within them help to increase fat utilisation, thereby 'sparing' precious glycogen. Of course, there's another important strategy to help us avoid running out of energy, and that's taking carbs on board during the run, which we'll cover in detail in Section 6.

## Fatigue–resistant muscles

Muscular endurance refers to the muscles' capacity to make repeated contractions for an extended period. Muscles are made up of thousands of cells, called fibres, of which there are distinct types with different attributes. 'Slow-twitch' fibres take time to reach their peak force and don't produce as much force as their 'fast-twitch' neighbours, but they are easy to recruit and very fatigue-resistant – perfect for logging lots of miles. In contrast, fast-twitch fibres can produce greater force and do so more rapidly – but they tire more quickly. Their 'crash and burn' nature means they are only recruited when a very high force output is required in a short amount of time – such as an explosive jump – or when the slow-twitch fibres' capacity has been exhausted through prolonged effort.

Unsurprisingly, elite distance runners tend to be endowed with a predominance of slow-twitch fibres, but the right kind of training can help any runner boost muscular endurance in three ways: 1) by making the existing slow-twitch fibres more fatigue-resistant, 2) by making some of the fast-twitch fibres (called 'type 2A fibres') behave more like slow-twitch fibres, and 3) by increasing the overall proportion of fibres that are recruited during exercise (akin to increasing the size of your workforce). This latter strategy involves something most runners don't associate with marathon training – sprinting. We'll look at how to incorporate this into marathon training in the next chapter.

## A robust musculoskeletal system

It's not just the cardiovascular system that needs staying power. The marathon runner's muscles, bones and connective tissues (the musculoskeletal system) also need to be able to 'endure' the demands placed upon them by prolonged high-impact exercise. Running itself will gradually build up your capacity to withstand the stresses, provided you progress your mileage slowly (both in terms of overall volume and long runs). Strength and conditioning also play a role in building a more bulletproof musculoskeletal system that is less susceptible to injury and able to recover from the rigours of training more quickly.

## The right mindset and psychological skills

You can be pretty sure that when Eliud Kipchoge ran the world's first sub-2-hr-marathon in 2019, he wasn't standing on the start line muttering 'I'll probably mess this up.' 'I bet I hit the wall.' Nor, when the going got really tough, did he let himself start thinking 'what's the point?' 'I feel awful...' In fact, he practised smiling at regular intervals, to lower his perception of effort. The point is that your mind isn't just a passenger on this marathon journey, it's the driver. In recent years, there's been compelling evidence regarding the true source of fatigue: not the body, but the mind. We'll be looking at techniques to improve mindset and focus as well as learning to become 'comfortable with being uncomfortable' in Chapter 6.

## Recovery capacity

The ability to bounce back from training quickly is a valuable asset for a marathoner. It's what enables you to maintain a high volume of training and handle numerous high-intensity sessions within your programme. But every runner's capacity for recovery is different, determined by genetics, age and experience, among other things. As you get fitter, your recovery will hasten a little – and you can help things along with some nutritional and lifestyle strategies that we'll look at in Chapter 9. But what's most important is getting to know how your body responds to training, so you can plan your schedule accordingly.

Feeling daunted by this lengthy list? Don't be. You will already be strong in some areas – others, you'll feel less confident about or maybe haven't even thought about before. The whole purpose of training is to get you from A (where you are now) to B (where you want to be). If you could already achieve your goal tomorrow, there'd be no need for it!

# How training works

In essence, developing fitness is a process of response and adaptation to training. When you place a training 'stress' (or 'load') on the body that slightly exceeds its current capacity, it is pushed outside its comfort zone. It responds to this stress by instigating the necessary adaptations within physiological, metabolic and musculoskeletal systems that will enable it to cope better next time. In other words, it becomes fitter.

There's a useful acronym for this: SAID – Specific Adaptation to Imposed Demands. What this means is that the training stress you place on your body needs to be *relevant* to what you are trying to achieve. For example, doing lots of swimming won't necessarily help you run quicker; the sort of training programme that might yield a Parkrun PB won't necessarily help your marathon campaign. This is known as 'training specificity'. It doesn't mean that every moment of physical activity that you do has to be running, nor that all your running must be at marathon pace – but it does have a bearing on what goes into your training programme, and when.

Another important issue is the magnitude of the training stress. If you add too much load at once, you overstress your body and risk injury, exhaustion or failing to complete, rather than adaptation. If you don't add enough, the stimulus isn't great enough to trigger adaptation. It's like the three bears' porridge in the fairy tale *Goldilocks* – it needs to be 'just right'.

As your body adapts to the 'imposed demands' though, the goalposts need to move. If you just carry on repeating the same thing, then what felt challenging in week three will be a breeze in week 10 and no longer create a training adaptation. That's why load needs to be progressive, in that it needs to get gradually more demanding as you get fitter, in order for you to continue gaining further training adaptations. This gradual increase in training stress is known as 'progressive overload'.

## Making progress

When we think of how to apply progressive overload, we tend to focus on volume (the total amount of 'work' being done, consisting of the number and length of the sessions you do). But bear in mind that increasing intensity (speed or effort) also adds to the overall training stress. Increasing both of them at once can inadvertently pile on too much overload at once, and this needs to be taken into account when structuring a training programme.

You may have heard of the '10 per cent rule': the notion that you should only increase your weekly training volume by 10 per cent at a time. It's not a bad guideline, but it won't be appropriate for everyone. For some, the progression will be unnecessarily slow and for others, too fast. The time when it should be most strictly abided by is when you are entering 'new territory' with your running, say, tackling runs that are significantly longer than you've done for a long time – or ever.

This ability to adapt to ever-increasing challenge is such a gift of the human body, especially the human body training for a marathon! It's why the idea of a 20-mile (32km) run with the last five at goal pace sounds preposterous right now but in a few months' time, will be thoroughly enjoyable. (OK, tolerable then!)

The other crucial factor in successful adaptation is recovery. The physiological adaptations don't take place when you're out there pounding the pavements and breaking a sweat – they happen when you are at rest. Building sufficient rest and recovery in to your plan ensures you'll get the maximum benefit from the hard work you put in. Following hard sessions with easy runs or rest days (the 'hard-easy rule') is the best way to balance training and recovery, though like all rules, it can sometimes be broken to achieve a particular aim (for example, preceding a long run with a fast workout to deliberately tire the legs and mimic the fatigue you'll feel in the late stages of a marathon).

A final principle to keep in mind is 'consistency'. As in not doing two weeks of intense training followed by two weeks during which you barely get out of the door. This seems to be one of the greatest challenges for marathon runners. It's partly because the training requirement is high (much higher than for shorter races), but it can also be due to poor plan structure (for example, you miss a session because you haven't left enough time to recover from the last one), a lack of organisation (you left your running shoes at work) or waning motivation. You can read more about making your training actually happen in Section 2.

In the next chapter, we'll look at the content and structure of marathon training in more detail.

# WHO IS THE AVERAGE MARATHON RUNNER?

The typical marathoner has changed drastically over the last few decades. Back in 1970, when the New York City marathon launched, the tiny field of 55 runners – all men – finished in an average time of 3 hrs 31 mins. By the end of the 1980s, the average finish time had slowed to just over 4 hrs, reflecting the fact that a wider range of people were taking part. A study of recreational marathon running worldwide between 2014–2017 by RunnerClick found that the average finish time for a man is now 4 hrs 13 mins and for a woman, 4 hrs 42 mins. More women are running marathons than ever before, with just under 35 per cent of marathoners being female. Age-wise, 61 per cent of marathon runners are between 30 and 49. My favourite stat of all? The fastest-growing age group participating in marathons in 2014–2017 was 90–99-year-olds!

# 2

# THE ART AND SCIENCE OF TRAINING

## The components and structure of a marathon plan

Let's get one thing straight. There is no single 'correct' way to train for a marathon. Even at the elite level, coaches and athletes approach the distance in different ways. These differences reflect attitudes and beliefs, training culture, role models, goals and experiences. It's not that the experts disagree about what they're trying to achieve, they just have different ideas on the best way of doing so.

The fact that a range of different approaches to marathon training can work illustrates another important point: we are all unique – what works best for one runner's body doesn't necessarily do the same for another. What worked for you at one time may not work for you now, or in the future, when your training status and experience level have changed. That's why it's so important to 'bring yourself into the equation' when considering your approach to training.

My own marathon-training philosophy has evolved over the years as a result of what I've learned from sport scientists and other coaches as well as my own personal marathon experiences and those of my clients.

The two biggest shifts in my thinking concern the structure of the training plan (what goes where) and the long runs – when to do them, how frequently and how fast.

While approaches may vary, there's little doubt that there is more to running a good marathon than logging lots of miles. You need a range of different training intensities to hone all those different fitness attributes outlined earlier. For example, low-intensity training improves fat utilisation, high-intensity running raises $VO_2$ max, and high mileage promotes running economy. All of these 'ingredients' should be part of your marathon-training recipe. What else is on the menu?

## Long runs

Every runner knows that long runs are the linchpin of marathon training. They are the most specific type of training session that you do to prepare for a marathon, which puts a tick in the 'specificity' box, while being on your feet for a long time helps build cardiovascular endurance as well as resilience within the musculoskeletal system. There's also an important psychological element – having to carry on running as fatigue builds improves mental strength and gives you the confidence that you can do it (even improving your capacity for tolerating the discomfort of doing so).

You'll need to get to grips with fuelling and hydrating on long runs – which is great preparation for the race itself. You can read more about how the gastrointestinal system adapts to fuelling through practice in Chapter 17 – but just as important is getting used to the practicalities of carrying fuel, and drinking on the move.

I mentioned that one of the shifts in my training philosophy related to long runs. Traditionally, marathon programmes include a weekly long run (with the odd break) that builds in distance week on week, culminating in the 'longest' long run, two to four weeks out from the race. Now, this doesn't really make sense. Why would you do your 'longest ever' run just a few weeks before your 'longest ever' race? Isn't that bunching up all the hard work too close together? How well are you going to recover between that peak run and the race? It's a lot better, I've found, to reach (or at least get close to) maximum long run distance much earlier in the programme (and revisit it occasionally), so

# THE LONG RUN - WHERE TO START AND HOW TO PROGRESS

When it comes to long runs, the word 'long' is relative. If you haven't run for longer than an hour in the last three months, then 75 minutes is going to be 'long' for you. If you run long most weekends, you might consider anything less than 15 miles (24.1km) a breeze.

The long runs in my training programmes begin at 12 miles (19.3km). I believe that you should already be comfortable running close to half-marathon distance from day one of your marathon-training programme. This enables the distance or duration to build at a manageable rate while giving you sufficient recovery.

Don't be disheartened if you're not there yet. Make building up weekly mileage and long-run distance your primary focus before you embark on a marathon plan. Your subsequent marathon experience will be much better for it.

How should you 'grow' your long run? Take the duration or distance of the longest run you've done in the previous four weeks as your starting point and add no more than 10 minutes or 1 mile (1.6km) to that. Build by 10 minutes or 1–2 miles (1.6–3.2km) each time you're ready to increase it. You don't have to add distance every week. There's nothing wrong with sticking to the same distance for a couple of long runs, or dropping down to a shorter distance sometimes. And having the odd break from long runs altogether is also fine – be it for rest, or for racing over a shorter distance, such as a 10K.

you can then switch the training focus to how *fast* you can run over a prolonged period.

The traditional marathon-training approach also assumes that if you don't do a long run virtually every week, you will somehow lose your ability to do it, which simply isn't true. Actually, it takes 21–28 days for your body to 'absorb' the benefits of a long run and instigate the adaptations it triggered. That's not to say that you need to have a gap of three to four weeks between long runs (running when you're tired is an important part of training – building 'fatigue resistance'). But I've found that most runners thrive better without the relentless grind of weekly, ever-longer long runs. *See* 'The long run – where to start and how to progress' on p. 27 for some advice on building your long run.

The practice of including some miles at goal marathon pace (or quicker than goal pace for runners whose marathon pace in itself isn't challenging) in long runs has become widespread in recent years. There are some really good reasons to do this. But remember, the first goal is to build up the run's duration. You want to be able to handle running 16–18 miles (25.7–29km) before worrying about going faster within the long run.

Once you reach that stage, adding in 'fast finishes' (the last few miles or minutes at a quicker pace), repeated bouts at marathon pace or runs that gradually progress from an easy pace to a quicker one will help you improve your marathon-specific endurance and you'll get better at resisting the fatigue that causes so many marathoners to slow down in the latter stages of the race.

## Lactate threshold training

The lactate threshold (LT) is the exercise intensity at which the accumulation of lactate starts to rise sharply. If you imagine a graph, with blood lactate levels on the y axis and running intensity (or speed) along the x axis, the goal of LT training is to push the LT further to the right. Training close to the pace/intensity associated with the LT has been shown to be an effective way of doing this, ultimately enabling you to maintain a higher speed without crossing the threshold and experiencing the negative effects it causes within the muscles.

Without wanting to muddy the waters, training at lactate threshold pace can also improve other variables, such as $VO_2$ max and running economy, which illustrates the point that training at any particular intensity level or speed affects the body as a whole, not just one specific physiological parameter. The idea that you must be training at intensity 'A' for one benefit and intensity 'B' for another, with anything in between being a sort of 'no man's land' is misleading. Yes, certain training intensities seem to do a good job of eliciting specific training effects, but ultimately the goal is to run a marathon faster, not to see your LT or $VO_2$ max score go up.

Back to lactate threshold training, then: first you need to know what your lactate threshold pace is and how running at it should feel. It is possible to have your lactate threshold measured in a lab – regular tiny blood samples are taken from your earlobe or fingertip while you run on a treadmill and the level of lactate is measured in relation to pace until you reach threshold. But unless you're going to repeat the measurement regularly, this can only provide a snapshot of where you are at that particular time. As your training advances, your LT – and the pace that it corresponds to – will improve. That's why going by 'feel' can be so useful, either on its own or as an adjunct to pace or heart rate. You can read more about how to monitor your effort level and intensity in Chapter 4.

But there are some other easy ways of figuring out where your lactate threshold falls. Sports scientists tell us that LT typically corresponds to the pace that a runner can maintain under race conditions for about an hour. For some runners, this means it will correspond to 10K race pace, but for others it'll be a little slower than 10K pace – around 15K or 10-mile race pace. But suffice to say it is NOT all-out effort. 'Comfortably hard' or 'controlled discomfort' are common descriptions of how this effort level should feel. It's likely to elicit a heart rate of 82–90 per cent of maximum.

In terms of training sessions, you'll be relieved to hear that running as fast as you can for an hour is not necessary! Continuous runs of 20–40 minutes (tempo runs) at a pace or effort level that is a tad lower than the LT can be alternated with long intervals (such as 6–10-minute reps) with relatively short recoveries performed at a pace (or effort level) that is slightly above it. I also like 'Unders and Overs' – a session in which you alternate short bouts of the two (faster than and slower than lactate threshold pace). This helps to improve your body's capacity for recycling the lactate that's been produced to use as an energy source.

## Speedwork

Speedwork is sometimes defined as training intended to improve your $VO_2$ max. I'm using the term more broadly here, to cover anything from maximal sprinting to intervals performed at, say, mile pace, 5K or 10K pace. This is because improving VO$_2$ max isn't our sole aim with faster sessions. It's been shown that VO$_2$ max can improve without a knock-on benefit to endurance performance and conversely, endurance performance can improve without a concomitant improvement in VO$_2$ max.

Whether it improves your VO$_2$ max or not, speed training is likely to benefit your running economy, muscle recruitment, neuromuscular efficiency (the line of communication between the brain and the muscles) and running form, as well as making submaximal speeds (including marathon pace) feel easier.

At the fastest end of the speed spectrum is maximal-pace running – sprinting. You may be sceptical about how this is going to improve your marathon prowess, and I hear you. Let's go back to those muscle fibres. The average distance runner rarely troubles their fast-twitch fibres because the forces of submaximal running aren't high enough to require them to be activated. But training the fast-twitch fibres means that when a high force is needed quickly – such as to make it up a steep hill, or produce a kick – you have a back-up team waiting in the wings. There is an even more compelling reason, though: when the slow-twitch fibres' capacity has been exhausted through prolonged effort (hello, mile 18/ kilometre 29!), these fibres can step in to share the workload with their knackered colleagues.

My programmes use the concept of the 'speed base', which I have borrowed from the US performance coach Steve Magness. Magness proposes that just as you need to build a foundation of endurance through running lots of easy miles, you need to build a foundation of speed through maximal speedwork. As marathon training advances, speedwork shifts, first to traditional intervals (corresponding closely to VO$_2$ max speed, or the maximum pace that could be maintained for around 6–9 minutes) and then to slower, but longer, reps (5K and 10K pace), which challenge your body in a way that more closely approximates the demands placed upon it by the marathon. One of the greatest benefits of this approach is that while you are focusing on building up your long run and overall weekly mileage in the first few weeks of training, the speedwork that sits alongside it – while very high in intensity – is extremely low in volume and does not drain your energy.

## A word about hills

YOU'LL OFTEN SEE the terms 'hill training' or 'hill reps'. Without context, these are rather vague – since 10-second hill sprints will have a very different training effect than will 60-second repetitions or a continuous tempo run on a hilly route.

Hills subtly change the demand of a run because you have to overcome gravity to get up them, increasing the load on your cardiovascular system and engaging more muscle fibres, building leg strength. (A less steep hill puts the emphasis more on speed while a steeper hill focuses more on strength development.) Like speedwork, the focus of hill training changes throughout the marathon-training cycle to meet the demands of training at that particular time. Read more about running on hills in Chapter 5.

## Easy and steady runs

I saved the best – and arguably most important – type of running session until last! Easy (aerobic) runs are the distance runner's bread and butter. Even at the elite level, the lion's share of training miles take place at a relatively low intensity. Why? Because this is what enables a runner to maintain a high volume of training. Studies show that upping mileage can translate to improved performance even when physiological parameters like $VO_2$ max don't change.

There's a continuum, of course, from a very easy 'I could do this all day' pace to a slightly more breathless, but still conversational, pace. When you are in the early stages of building mileage, it's sensible to focus on the easier end of the range. This enables you to increase volume without undue fatigue and with minimal injury risk. Easy-paced running also improves fat utilisation, increases capillarisation and, as you learned in Chapter 1, running lots helps to improve your running economy, so you can utilise oxygen more efficiently.

# How easy is 'easy'?

The most important determinant of an easy run is that it *feels* easy to you. If you tend to start easy runs at a faster pace than you end up finishing them, it's a hint that you're going too quick.

Often, target paces are suggested for easy runs that are related to your goal marathon pace. For example, you might be advised to run '25 per cent slower than marathon pace' or '90 seconds slower than marathon pace'. This guideline can work OK for quicker runners (sub-3 hrs 30 mins, as a guideline) because their marathon pace is likely to be at a higher percentage of their maximum capacity, relatively speaking, than a slower runner's marathon pace. Their easy runs will certainly need to be slower than marathon pace, because marathon pace will not feel 'easy'. But less swift runners often find that goal marathon pace *does* feel easy – or that they can run a little quicker than their goal marathon pace during easy runs. It's that extrapolation problem again (*see* Introduction).

Let's take an example. A speedy runner aiming to maintain 7-minute-miling (4 mins 20 secs per km) on race day would be looking at easy runs of 8 mins 45 secs per mile (5 mins 26 secs per km) or thereabouts to tick the '25 per cent slower' box. But a runner aiming for 10 mins per mile (6 mins 12 secs per km) on the day would be prescribed easy runs at 12 mins 30 secs per mile (7 mins 46 secs per km) pace, which is likely to feel more like a trudge and result in poor technique and shuffling.

That's why I recommend going by feel (heart rate can also be a useful tool) as well as checking that your pace remains relatively consistent throughout the run. Read more about monitoring the intensity of your runs in Chapter 4.

# Going steady

When you are more into the swing of marathon training, and more comfortable with handling a higher weekly mileage, some of your easy runs can get a little quicker – described as 'steady' runs. In my experience, many people mistakenly perform their easy runs at this slightly quicker pace as a matter of course. Try not to make all your easy runs steady, as it will make the task of building your endurance base unnecessarily hard. Steady runs are often defined in relation to marathon pace – 30 seconds slower per mile (1.6km), or 5–10 per cent slower, than goal marathon pace, for example. But again, this won't necessarily hold true for less speedy runners who may find that their steady run pace is actually perfectly aligned with their marathon pace, or even a little quicker.

## Putting a plan together

So you've got the ingredients – what's the recipe? How are you going to fit all these different types of session into a plan, without overwhelming the body with too many training stresses at once? Let's talk about 'periodisation'.

This is the concept of breaking down training into distinct periods or phases, each with a specific focus. Terms like 'mesocycle' and 'microcycle' are used to describe different-length blocks of training that make up the whole – but the important thing is that the focus of training shifts as you go along. This isn't about doing *more* training, it's about the *type* of training you do.

Originally, periodisation was seen as a set of discrete stages – each different phase followed on from the one before. For example, a base endurance phase, followed by a strength phase, a speed endurance phase... But then some coaches began to wonder, if all of these aspects of fitness are important for the marathon, won't laying one aside while you focus on another allow the gains achieved to tail off? This led to a slightly different approach to periodisation.

In 'non-linear' periodisation, you don't disregard any aspect of fitness that you've already developed. It takes less input to *maintain* a component of fitness than it does to develop it in the first place, so including a small amount of training at a range of different intensities *alongside* your main training focus allows you to keep on top of things. It's akin to a juggler keeping all their balls in the air.

I've found this to be an effective way of addressing all the necessary fitness requisites of marathon training without overloading a runner. It also makes the plan more varied and less monotonous. Balance is key, of course. It's not about trying to improve everything at once.

This is the method I've used to devise the six marathon programmes in this book. While they differ in volume and, to a lesser degree, content, they all progress through the same main phases of training, which are outlined over the page. There is more detailed information on each training plan in Section 2.

# TRAINING PHASES - AS EASY AS 1, 2, 3

## 1. The Foundation phase - building a base

The first priority for a marathon is to build a good aerobic or endurance base – this is the foundation on which we'll later lay the stones of more specific training. Building an endurance base is about volume (remember, volume refers to the amount of training rather than intensity). Runs are performed at a pace that is manageable and comfortable, so that you can a) continue for long enough and b) repeat often.

The endurance base prepares you to handle a high volume of running. 'High' is a relative term, though. If you are an elite athlete, high could mean 125 miles (200km) a week or more. I don't recommend this! On the other hand, racing 26.2 miles (42.2km) is going to be a big ask if you have never exceeded 20 miles (32km) a week in training. I don't concur with coaches who state that to run a good marathon, you must be running 50 or 60 or 70 miles (80, 97 or 113km) a week. In fact, I've often found that runners

attempting this (alongside busy family lives and jobs) actually do better when they *reduce* their mileage. But let's be realistic and acknowledge that you need to include sufficient mileage on a consistent basis. I've allowed a longer Foundation phase in my first-timer programmes, because less experienced runners are less likely to have already established a strong base.

So what else goes into the Foundation phase? Well, with our focus on building volume, it'd be foolish to throw in lots of demanding interval work and lactate threshold training at the same time (though this is exactly what many marathon programmes do). But you can include small amounts of high-intensity – almost maximal – work, which serves as a foundation for subsequent speedwork (as discussed on p. 30) and gives your body a novel training stimulus without adding much additional load.

The sprint training I've included in the programmes isn't aerobic, so it isn't about improving your aerobic energy system, VO$_2$ max or lactate threshold. Instead, the onus is on improving the efficiency of the neuromuscular system. This will not only contribute to the activation of a greater percentage of muscle fibres, but also increase the speed at which your brain sends signals to the muscles, making you run more efficiently and economically.

The Foundation phase is also a good time to introduce some strength and conditioning work, if you aren't already doing some. This will help to improve your resistance to injury and fatigue as marathon training progresses. *See* Chapter 11 for more on getting stronger.

## 2. The Development phase – building endurance and speed

By the time you transition into the Development phase, your running volume will be close to its peak, as will your long run distance. The aim is to maintain it (which, you'll be relieved to be reminded, doesn't require as much input as building it in the first place). This means you won't be doing increasingly longer long runs week in, week out, freeing up some capacity to develop the intensity of some of your other runs with the goal of improving your ability to sustain pace over distance.

This phase is where you'll find more of those 'slightly-harder-than-easy' steady runs and lactate threshold training featuring in the plan. By nudging your lactate threshold upwards, remember, you'll be able to maintain a higher proportion of your maximal capacity during prolonged running.

The focus of speedwork also shifts in the Development phase, moving away from maximal-intensity sprints and towards interval training at intensities ranging from VO$_2$ max (which typically equates to the best pace you could run 1–2 miles/1.6–3.2km at) to 5K and 10K pace. There'll also be some hill training to develop strength and speed endurance and to vary the biomechanical effort from flat terrain. Not wanting to let go of what we've already achieved, we'll still be 'checking in' with base speed every now and again during the Development phase, through hill or flat sprints and strides.

### 3. The Specific phase – honing in on marathon pace

This next phase is all about specificity – the aim is to improve your capacity to resist fatigue at marathon pace. Physiologically speaking, it's about how well you can resist the declines in lactate threshold, oxygen uptake and running economy that accompany fatigue.

Some of your long runs now become more focused – not just easy miles, but bouts of running at race pace, or long runs that start easy but finish hard. Shorter runs at paces that are close to goal pace are also valuable – helping you maximise efficiency at that particular pace and strengthening your 'feel' for the right pace so that you are less likely to make costly pacing errors on race day.

A 'dress rehearsal' (NOT of 26.2 miles/42.2km!) is a really important run to include a few weeks out from race day. Run it on the same sort of terrain you'll be racing on, ideally at the same time of day, and make sure it includes some marathon pace mileage. Perhaps the most valuable benefit of this run is in building confidence, but it also serves as an advance warning system about anything that isn't going right. For example, perhaps your proposed fuelling strategy isn't delivering the goods. Or the socks you were going to wear give you blisters. There's more information on scheduling a dress rehearsal in 'The Programmes' section.

Of course, the specific phase isn't exclusively about marathon pace. You still want to maintain the speed and strength endurance built earlier in the plan, and you can do this with lower-volume workouts that won't contribute to excessive fatigue.

### 4. The Taper phase – winding down

The final phase of training is the taper or 'winding down' period (*see* Chapter 15). Here, the focus switches from training to recovery, from gaining fitness to consolidating those gains.

# The role of cross-training

It might sound odd for me to say that cross-training can play a valuable role in your marathon programme, given the principle of specificity outlined in Chapter 1.

But alternatives to running, like cycling, elliptical training or rowing, can add to (or help you maintain) your training load, while non-cardio activities like yoga and Pilates can bring balance, supporting and complementing your running.

Why not just run more? Maybe you've learned from past experience that high mileage raises your own personal injury risk. A weekly bike ride or swim could provide an additional cardiovascular workout without increasing the load on your joints. Perhaps you just want more variety – in which case you could swap an easy run for an exercise class, or substitute a long run with a mid-length run followed by a bike ride, which would reduce the volume of running while still maintaining the overall duration of the workout.

Don't see cross-training as a way of upping your training, just because you think 'more is better' though. It still forms part of your overall training volume, even though it isn't running, and can therefore deplete glycogen, create muscle damage and fatigue and require recovery. During marathon training, you are almost certainly going to be running more than usual already, so trying to swim, hit the gym and cycle on other days may tip the balance too far. This is particularly true if the cross-training activity you are introducing is one that your body is not accustomed to. Swimming might sound less stressful on the body than running, but if you haven't been for a decade then 50 laps of the pool is likely to be pretty exhausting!

As useful as cross-training can be, it's not a 'like-for-like' substitute. Your heart and lungs may not have a clue what type of activity you are doing, but your nervous system – which governs muscle fibre recruitment and hones your movement efficiency – certainly does. That's why specificity is one of the principles of training – and why running is the best training for runners.

## Cross-training through injury

One situation in which judicious use of cross-training can enable you to maintain, or even gain, fitness is when you are managing a niggle, or coming back from injury. You may be able to run a little, but not enough for marathon training, so you can supplement this with cross-training to help you build volume without overdoing things.

Even if you can't run at all, cardiovascular cross-training can help you minimise fitness losses. The best activity to do is the one that causes no pain to your injured area, so you will need to test out different options to see what feels right. One of the most effective, and least impactful, options is aqua running. (*See* 'Walking on water'). Cycling, walking, swimming and cardio machines, such as the rower or elliptical trainer, are other good options.

## Walking on water

AQUAJOGGING IS OFTEN described as the 'best' form of cross-training for runners, because the biomechanics are so similar to running on land. It can be as aerobically challenging, too, because water has 12 times the resistance of air.

- CONSIDER USING A buoyancy belt, which is secured around your hips to keep you higher in the water. (You can do it without, too.)

- THE WATER MUST be deep enough for you to move your legs without touching the bottom of the pool.

- REMEMBER TO USE your arms in a running motion rather than a treading water action.

- AIM FOR A leg turnover of roughly half your land leg turnover speed (for instance, if your cadence is usually 180spm, aim for 90spm).

- DON'T LEAN FORWARDS – stay upright.

- BUILD IN SOME breaks on your first few attempts – this is tough training, so go for 3–5-minute bouts with a 30–60-second recovery in between – 15–20 minutes in total is sufficient to start with.

- Replicate your running sessions, rather than just paddling monotonously at the same intensity for the same duration each time.

I once coached someone who developed shin splints midway through marathon training. We moved all his training to the stationary bike and pool, simulating (or adapting) the planned running workout to the cross-training activity. For example, if a session was geared towards improving lactate threshold, he did long intervals at a 'comfortably hard' effort with short recoveries. If it was speedwork, intervals of aquajogging as hard as possible, interspersed with gently treading water, fitted the bill. Hills were replicated by pushing a heavy gear on the bike, or standing out of the saddle. He still achieved his sub-3 hrs 30 mins goal in the marathon.

## Complementing your running

Cross-training can also play a supportive or complementary role to your running. Activities like yoga and Pilates – as well as strength training (check out the Foundation Plan and Performance Plan in Chapter 11) – fit in here. They provide balance to your programme and address some of the physical qualities that running doesn't develop, such as good posture, balance, core strength and mobility.

People often ask when to do these activities. On rest days? After running? The answer depends on how challenging and intense the activity is. I would generally expect this type of cross-training to be low-intensity and therefore, it doesn't much matter when you do it. But strength training with weights would be the exception. You can read more about where to fit strength training into your schedule in Chapter 11.

Ultimately, the best way to determine whether to include cross-training in your marathon-training plan is to ask yourself what purpose it will serve. It needs to be there for a reason (even if that reason is simply because you enjoy a weekly swim or exercise class), or you risk simply adding to the stress that running is already placing on your body.

# DOUBLING UP

'Double days' are days on which you run twice. Elite runners use them to increase their overall training volume. Should you? It depends. If you have two or more non-running days per week, you might be best off adding a run to one of those days to increase volume, rather than doubling up on an existing training day. Unless, that is, it's actually easier for you to do so on a practical level – for example, if you run commute. There's also some evidence that double days offer 'two bites of the cherry' in terms of the physiological response to training. One study found that training twice a day, every other day, improved endurance capacity more than did daily training – though other research found that although many training parameters improved, this did not translate to better performance.

One way you can use a double day is as an alternative to lengthening a single run (excepting the long run) to the point that it becomes 'too long' in terms of your time or energy availability. Two 4-mile (6.4km) runs are less depleting than one 8-mile (12.8km) run, even though both add the same amount to your overall weekly mileage. That said, part of the purpose of training is to create a certain amount of fatigue, which then leads to adaptation, so splitting runs into two to escape getting tired isn't necessarily always a good option, especially when it comes to long runs.

# 3
# ALL ABOUT YOU

## Determining your starting point and goal

We've looked in detail at the demands of the marathon and the nuts and bolts of a marathon-training plan. But where do you, the runner, fit into all this? I would hope you have – at some point – stood on a race start line, whether it be a 10K or a previous marathon. (And if you haven't, make sure you take part in a few other races before taking on the marathon.) But that still leaves a potentially very diverse range of runners who could be reading this book. You could have been running for two years, or 12 years. You could be a 25-year-old woman, or a 59-year-old man. Perhaps you run three times a week, perhaps six. Maybe you've never had an injury, maybe you have the physio under Favourites on your phone. . .

This is important, because the training priorities will be different for an experienced runner looking to shave time off a PB than for someone who is tackling the distance for the first time. Coaches talk about 'chronological age' and 'training age'. The latter refers to how long someone has been actively training in their sport – so two runners could share the same birthday but still have a very different training age, and therefore respond to – and cope with – training very differently.

Training priorities also vary according to personal strengths and weaknesses – for example, a real 'endurance monster' versus someone who runs a great 5K but struggles with long runs and high weekly mileage. That's why the marathon programmes I've created for this book are not time-based (e.g. 'the sub-4 hour plan') but based on experience level and training volume. It's also why I keep harping on about bringing yourself into the training equation.

## Know thyself

An honest appraisal of your 'running life' (your history, strengths and weaknesses) is crucial as you embark on this – your first or next – marathon journey, helping to determine both your starting point and the path your training follows. Consider the following questions – you may want to note down your answers as they could affect decisions you make about your training:

- How long have you been running? (Training age)
- How old are you? (Chronological age)
- Do you get injuries frequently, and is there any indication as to what triggers injuries for you?
- How much do you currently run each week and how consistent are you? (A good tip to help you work this out is to add up the last six weeks' mileage and divide it by six. Does this figure tally with what you would have said was your typical weekly volume? We're often less consistent than we like to think!)
- Have you run a marathon before?
- If so, what went well, what went less well?
- If not, what is the furthest distance you have run and how did it feel?
- What type of runs do you most look forward to? Which ones do you dread? (This tends to fall in with where our natural strengths and weaknesses lie.)

## How committed are you?

There's another factor to consider that's quite separate from your previous experiences and strengths and weaknesses: your willingness –

and ability – to commit to a sustained period of training. This isn't just about motivation but practicality. For example, perhaps you're absolutely determined not to forfeit your place in the London marathon, but you've got a young baby. Or you've secured a charity place, but you're still rehabbing from a long-standing injury. Or you're aiming to achieve a Good for Age standard but there's a big work project eating up all your spare time...

These real-life issues can't be ignored. There are – and always will be – 24 hours in a day. So, when you begin marathon training, the hours you spend running (and on supporting activities) will be replacing hours that you previously spent doing something else. I'm not suggesting that you must devote your entire life to marathon training, seven days a week, for the next few months. But if you can't realistically fit in even three or four days a week on a regular basis, the chances are you won't achieve the fitness level that will allow you to do the marathon justice.

Here are some more questions to consider:

- How much time each week are you willing and able to commit to training for the marathon?
- Is your finish time important to you?
- Are there any major obstacles or commitments in your life between now and the race that may conflict with your training?
- What do(es) your family/partner feel about you running the marathon? It's really helpful to have their support, be it practical or emotional.
- Have you got long enough to prepare for the race you have in mind in a way that you'll be satisfied with?

## The ticking clock

People often ask 'How long do I need to train for a marathon?' The answer is, it depends. If you're already running 30-plus miles (50km-plus) a week and regularly do half-marathons, you could hit the ground running (excuse the pun) on day one of a 12-week marathon-training programme with high aspirations. But if you're nowhere near that point, then you may need to make time, in effect, to 'get fit' for your marathon programme. If you don't, then the slope you'll have to climb, in terms of training intensity, will be very steep and the risk of injury or burnout high (unless you choose to set your sights lower – focusing on completing, rather than competing, this time around).

Instead of saying everyone should allow X amount of time to build up to a marathon, I prefer to say that everyone should be comfortable running 12–13 miles (19–20km) and clocking up 20–25 (32–40km) miles per week by the time they start their specific build-up (such as one of my 20-week programmes) for the race.

If that leaves you wanting to throw this book across the room, take heart. It's not that running a marathon isn't possible without these prerequisites, it's just that my experience shows me that if you need to spend the first few weeks of a training plan getting comfortable running above 10 miles (16km), you won't be left with long enough to progress to where you need to be before the race. This doesn't mean that you can't follow one of my programmes – but I'd advise allowing a few extra weeks beforehand to build up your training volume to an appropriate level before you embark on one of them. *See* 'The long run – where to start and how to progress' on p. 27 for advice on how to build up your training volume.

## Going for goals

So what time are you thinking you'd like to run this marathon in? I find runners come in two varieties – those who 'just want to finish' and those who want to run 'sub-something' (sub-3 hrs, sub-3 hrs 45 mins, sub-4 hrs 30 mins etc).

To the first group, I say this. While I understand the sentiment, the vagueness of this statement isn't all that helpful because it means there's no specific focus or direction for your training. What sort of sessions should you do? What pace or effort level will be appropriate for your long runs? Frankly, if you really just 'want to finish', you could probably crawl around the course next week if you really had to. It's more likely that you want to finish without too much agony, and ideally with a smile on your face. So, while the type and amount of training you do may be different from a PB-hungry veteran, it's still important to have at least an idea of what you can realistically achieve or would be happy with. (*See* 'Why do I need a goal time?' over the page, for more information.)

# WHY DO I NEED A GOAL TIME?

Having a goal time allows you to work out the associated goal pace ('marathon pace' or 'race pace'). For example, completing in 3 hrs 30 mins requires an average goal pace of 8 mins per mile (4 mins 58 secs per km). That does not mean that you should be doing all your training sessions, including long runs, at 8 mins per mile pace, but it is definitely sensible to include some training at goal pace, so that you become familiar with how it feels and can 'lock on' to it quickly come race day. It is also useful as a basis for setting appropriate paces (both quicker and slower) for other training sessions.

As far as runners with specific time targets are concerned, it sounds obvious, but you can't just pluck your desired goal out of nowhere. A lot of runners do this – they tell me they'd like a 'sub-4' as if it's a product that can be selected from a supermarket shelf. Your goal time needs to be evidence-based and grounded in reality.

## Figuring out your potential

The first port of call is to look at your existing (previous) race times, to see what they suggest you are capable of running in a marathon.

If you're a first-timer, but you've run a half-marathon, the simplest starting point is to multiply your half-marathon time by two and add 10–20 minutes. But you'll get a broader picture by using one of the many online 'race prediction' calculators. These use algorithms to predict one race-distance time from another (by estimating how much faster or slower you'd be over the shorter or longer distance).

If you've already got a marathon or two (or few) under your belt, factor this in to your considerations. How accurate were any time predictions you made on those occasions? Are you more or less fit since then?

The advantage of using race prediction calculators is that you can plug in times from a variety of different race distances – this gives you a hint about where your strengths and weaknesses lie. For example, let's say your 5K time predicts you can run a marathon in 3 hrs 12 mins but your half-marathon time predicts 3 hrs 29 mins – that suggests you are stronger over shorter distances and will need to focus heavily on building endurance and stamina. I'd be advising you to set your goal closer to the 3 hrs 29 mins than 3 hrs 12 mins!

Bear in mind, though, that the less similar the race distance you are using to predict from is to the marathon distance, the less accurate it is likely to be. For example, predicting your marathon potential from a 20-mile (32km) race is more insightful than doing it from a 1-mile (1.6km) time. My modus operandi is to feed in as many recent race times as possible to establish a 'range of potential'.

You need to consider terrain, too – did you achieve the race time you are basing your prediction on in a race over similar terrain to the marathon? Or was it through blanket bog? And when was the race you're predicting from? Don't use ancient times that no longer represent your current level of fitness.

I use the McMillan Running Pace Calculator (an excellent – and currently free – resource) for my own training and coaching and find it very accurate in predicting shorter distances – such as a half-marathon time from a 10K. But I find it consistently overambitious in predicting a marathon time from a half-marathon time, particularly with non-elite runners. So I'll note down what it says, but take it with a big pinch of salt.

Remember, these calculators aren't perfect. They are formulaic predictions. How can they know that you are an endurance fiend, who gets stronger the longer you go? Or that you've only ever run two 5Ks? View them as a helpful tool, rather than the be-all and end-all.

Once you have an idea of what is achievable 'on paper', go back to those two sets of questions on p. 42 and p. 43. Factoring in your answers will help you fine-tune your goal and decide whether to 'dream big' or settle for a less aggressive goal for this particular marathon (especially if it's your debut). It's worth noting that very few people run their best ever marathon on their first go – see it as putting down a marker, rather than as a one-off opportunity, and take comfort in the fact that it will be a PB whatever the clock says.

## Monitor and review

Even after you have decided on your marathon goal and embarked on a training programme to reach it, don't feel that it is set in stone. Monitoring your progress as the weeks go by will allow you to decide whether you want to modify your goal up or down. This doesn't only mean judging yourself on mid-term race performances – it also involves keeping tabs on how you *feel*. How are you recovering from long runs? Are you developing niggles? Do you feel tired all the time?

Keeping a training journal is a great way of monitoring how you are responding to your training plan (there are other benefits, too, which you can read about on p. 61). The coaching platform Final Surge asks you to rate not just how hard you felt the session was (on a scale of 1 to 10) but also how good you felt. I think this is an important distinction. Training isn't necessarily going to feel easy but you want to be feeling good, not despondent and exhausted. I recommend using a similar system in your own training log.

# 4

# MONITORING YOUR TRAINING

## How to keep tabs on your efforts

You are going to be working at various different levels of intensity during marathon training. How will you monitor your efforts? What should your heart rate be at lactate threshold? What pace should your 'easy' runs be at?

We runners are spoilt for choice when it comes to tech that monitors and measures what our bodies are doing in training. We can check heart rate, pace, calorie expenditure and even power output with smart watches and other gadgets. But doing so is not essential. For the hundreds of years before this kind of technology was available, people ran by feel. *Does it feel easy? Can I keep this effort level going for the next two hours?* OK, so I'm a Luddite. Don't worry, I'm not suggesting you throw out your tech – I use it myself. But I do think it is incredibly important to be able to gauge your effort level and pace without relying on external feedback.

## Listening to your body

There are two commonly used tech-free methods of 'rating' how hard you are working: 1) the rate of perceived exertion (RPE) scale and 2) the 'talk' test.

## Rating effort

To monitor your exercise intensity using RPE you simply need to ask yourself 'how hard am I working?' and rate it on a scale. The classic 'Borg' scale (named after its founder), which is often used in science lab performance testing, ranges from 6 (no exertion) to 20 (maximal exertion). A simpler, modified Borg scale ranges from 0 (nothing at all) to 10 (maximum). But really, it doesn't matter what scale you use as long as you have a way of rating how much effort you are putting in and an understanding of how much effort you are *meant* to be putting in to achieve the desired training stimulus of that particular session. For example, if you are doing a tempo run and it's meant to feel like a 7 out of 10 effort, but you feel it's a 9, then you need to ease off.

One of the advantages of using an intuitive method of rating effort, rather than an absolute one, like pace, is that it is adaptable and responsive. I often find that people get very hung up on hitting specific paces, without taking into account the factors that might affect it. If you were doing that tempo run on a flat, level tarmac surface with no wind, then the goal pace of, say, 8-minute-miling (4 mins 58 secs per km), might be achievable – and elicit a 7 out of 10 effort rating. But factor in a headwind, a very hot day or a knobbly trail, and trying to maintain 8-minute-miling is now pushing your RPE too high.

It might all sound a little unscientific – especially to technophiles – but studies have found that RPE tallies well with oxygen uptake and heart rate. In other words, our inbuilt ability to assess how hard we're working is remarkably accurate (in adults at least – less so for kids).

## We need to talk

Another zero-tech method of gauging effort is the Talk Test. Here, rather than rating how hard you're working on a scale, you're measuring it against how much – or little – conversation you can get out. For example, on easy runs, you should feel comfortable chatting to a companion. On a tempo run, you should only have enough breath to utter the odd phrase.

The Talk Test and RPE have another plus point: they allow for daily fluctuations in your energy levels and performance. Your 'somewhat easy' effort on a day that you're feeling good might see you averaging 9 mins 30 secs per mile (5 mins 54 secs per km), while on a more fatigued or stressed day, you might only manage 9 mins 50 secs per mile. If you were to be working solely with pace, trying to achieve 9 mins 30 secs pace might take you out of the 'somewhat easy' zone where you were meant to be working.

## FACTORS AFFECTING RPE

Anything from a bad night's sleep to dehydration, a lack of food or the first hint of a cold can raise your sense of effort. I talk more about how time of day can affect your RPE in Chapter 5 (which will depend on whether you are a 'lark' or an 'owl') and offer advice on optimising recovery in Chapter 9.

Women may find that their sense of effort is affected by where they are in their menstrual cycle. One study found that women rated an exercise session as tougher when it was performed between days five and seven of their cycle (the first day of your menstrual bleed is considered to be day one, so this would likely be the tail-end of a period), compared to when it was performed in the mid-luteal phase, between days 19 and 21. Other research suggests that women perceive the 'best' time, performance wise, is just after bleeding has ceased (the late follicular phase). A review published in 2021 concluded that while there are not clear, consistent effects on specific measures of performance (such as strength or oxygen uptake) across the board, women consistently identify a drop in performance during the early follicular and late luteal phases. Research – woefully inadequate until now – continues. The best way of determining whether your energy levels and RPE ebb and flow at different times of the month is to record your menstrual cycle in your training diary and look for any patterns.

### Right on pace

All that said, I do use pace in my one-to-one coaching. When a runner has specific time goals they want to achieve, it's useful to be able to set pace guidelines for different training sessions, including runs (or sections of runs or intervals) at 'goal race pace'. It could be described as the only truly objective measure of performance – after all, if you need to be running 7-minute miles (4 mins 20 secs per km) to achieve your goal, it doesn't matter what your RPE or heart rate says – it's this pace or bust!

In training, however, I would always give a pace range, rather than a set figure, as a guideline. For example, 6 mins 55 secs–7 mins 10 secs per mile (4 mins 17 secs–4 mins 27 secs per km), rather than 7-minute-miling.

I don't 'prescribe' every run by pace. It can be stressful and dispiriting to feel chained to your watch, stripping the joy out of running as well as reducing your ability to judge pace using your own intuition and awareness. Rather than relying solely on this rigid parameter, I use it in conjunction with other methods of monitoring – and not for all types of run.

## From the heart

Heart rate monitoring is another option. The more effort you put into a run, the greater the number of times your heart has to beat per minute in order to pump blood to the working muscles, so it opens a window on how your physiology is responding to running. But while it's easy to glance at your sports watch and see that your heart is beating at, say, 150bpm, this fact on its own tells you nothing useful.

Is 150bpm 'good' or 'bad' – low or high? Where *should* your heart rate be during any particular session? Are you *meant* to be working hard during this particular run, or not? Heart rate needs context to be useful. That context usually comes from what percentage the figure represents of your maximum heart rate (MHR). Is 150bpm 72 per cent of your maximum – or 92 per cent?

### Working out maximum heart rate

A reminder of the standard formula for determining maximum heart rate: 220 minus your age. The age component reflects the fact that as we get older, our maximum heart rate decreases. Perhaps surprisingly, sedentary adults and active runners experience similar rates of declines in maximal heart rate as they get older, with a drop of approximately one beat per year. But that doesn't mean that 220 minus your age is an accurate reflection of your maximum – individuals vary, and your true maximum could be as many as 10 beats higher or lower than your age-predicted estimate.

An alternative formula that has been shown to be a little more reliable is 207 minus (0.7 x age) but again, it's only a guideline.

There are two ways of getting a more personalised and accurate measure. The first involves actually running at peak aerobic speed, either on the road or in the lab. In a $VO_2$ max test, you run as hard as you can (usually on a treadmill at increasing speed and gradient) until you reach exhaustion, while various physiological parameters are monitored. On the road, your heart rate during the last couple of minutes of an all-out 5K race will be a reasonable reflection of your max.

The second option doesn't involve maximal running. Instead, it introduces your resting heart rate (RHR) into the 220 minus your age equation, allowing you to calculate what your heart rate should be at different levels of effort with more accuracy.

## The heart rate reserve method

Resting heart rate, as it says on the tin, is the number of times your heart beats per minute when you are fully at rest. As such, it should be measured first thing in the morning, ideally in bed and definitely before caffeine! If you don't have a watch that measures heart rate, simply place your index and middle fingers on the underside of your opposite wrist and once you've detected your pulse, count how many times your heart beats in one minute.

RHR is influenced by fitness level (though there is a genetic component, too). A lower resting heart rate means that your body is delivering more oxygenated blood per beat and therefore can beat fewer times per minute than a heart that delivers less blood per beat. When your resting heart rate decreases, it's a sign that you have become fitter.

Armed with your age-predicted maximum heart rate and resting heart rate, the formula below (known as the Karvonen formula or Heart Rate Reserve method) enables you to calculate what your heart rate should be at different percentages of maximum effort:

Percentage of maximum required (%) = (MHR – RHR) x % + RHR

Let's take an example. Sarah is 38 years old. Her age-predicted MHR is therefore 182bpm. Her measured resting heart rate is 50bpm. Sarah wants to know what her heart rate should be on a tempo run, which her coach has told her should be run at around 85 per cent of her maximum heart rate. She also wants to know where it should be on easy runs, which she's read should be closer to 70 per cent of maximum.

*85% of MHR = (MHR – RHR) x 85% + RHR

85% = (182 – 50) x 85% + 50

85% = 132 x 85% = 112 + 50 = 162bpm

(*To work out what 70 per cent would be, simply repeat the formula with 70 per cent in place of 85 per cent.)

If Sarah had simply used the 220 minus age formula to work out what 85 per cent should be, she would have got a different answer:

220 – 38 = 182bpm

85% of 182 = 155bpm

This lower heart rate guideline reflects the fact that Sarah's resting heart rate – which is well below average, reflecting her fitness level – has not been factored into the equation.

I should stress that, like pace, heart rate guidelines should always be a range rather than a specific figure. In our example, Sarah might look at around 5 beats either side of 162bpm at 85 per cent or 'tempo' pace.

## And the winner is...

In my opinion, a combination of different methods of gauging intensity is better than any single measure. Let's say I have a coaching client whose preference is to work with heart rate. They are performing a tempo run at 85 per cent of MHR, which, according to the Karvonen formula, should be around 162bpm. However, at 162bpm, the runner cannot utter a single word and rates their effort level at 9 out of 10. Given that a tempo run is meant to feel 'comfortably hard', their level of effort at a heart rate of 162bpm is far too great, despite the fact that it appears to be 'correct'. In this scenario, I would get them to go by feel. What pace *feels* like a 7 out of 10 effort? What *feels* comfortably hard?

The same holds true for pace. A training pace calculator might have told you that your 'easy runs' should be at 9-minute-miling. But say it turns out that 9-minute-miling doesn't feel easy to you – 10-minute-miling does.

What do you do? For me, the answer would be listen to your body and be responsive to what it is telling you.

Devices are a great way of gathering feedback – and keeping track of your mileage/time spent running. They can also be motivational – a new record for longest run or fastest mile brings joy to any runner. But don't become a slave to your gadgets.

The Monitoring Intensity table in Appendix 2 on pp. 278–9 gathers together many different ways of determining and measuring the effort level for different types of session to give you a range of ways of checking that you are in the right ballpark for that particular type of session. Using this table will help you improve your awareness of what different types of run in the marathon programmes should feel like, which in turn will help you utilise pace and heart rate in a more flexible way.

# THE MARATHON PROGRAMMES

This section introduces the marathon-training plans. While you can follow one of them even if you haven't read the rest of the book, to understand the science underpinning the programmes, you should read Chapters 1 and 2. And when deciding which programme is most suitable for your current level of experience and aspiration, I recommend reading Chapter 3.

There are six programmes in total – with two levels of experience ('First-timer' and 'Experienced') within each of three categories.

If you are a marathon novice, I recommend you follow the First-timer option of your chosen programme, even if you have been running for a while. The 'building' phase – the 'Foundation' – lasts eight weeks on these plans. You might also choose this option if you consider yourself prone to running injuries, or even if you've run a marathon before, but it did not go to plan. For more seasoned marathoners, the Experienced level is likely to be more appropriate. This allows a six-week Foundation phase and longer Developmental and Specific training phases. (*See* pages 34–6 for a reminder of the different training phases.) But do use your gut feeling alongside logic. If one plan 'feels' more right for you than the other, it might suit you better.

The three categories are defined by training volume and load.

- The **'Full Throttle'** plans typically entail five days' training per week and are the highest in volume.
- The **'Steady State'** plans are a little less demanding on your time (typically four days' training per week, with the odd five-day week) but the intensity level is similar.
- In the **'Minimalist'** plans, both the volume and intensity are lower (because to maintain the same level of intensity the programme would be skewed too far towards speed rather than endurance). These plans require three or four training days per week.

All the programmes are 20 weeks in length and require you – first-timer or not – to be *comfortable* running 12–13 miles (19.3–20.9km) from the outset. (When I say comfortable, I mean it should be something you are already doing semi-regularly, not something you've managed once.) As I explain on p. 27, I believe this is a sensible prerequisite for anyone embarking on marathon training.

If you look at the amount of training involved in any particular programme and see that it's way beyond what you've done previously, consider choosing one with less volume, even if you have the time and motivation to do the more challenging one. Yes, you need to be challenging yourself to trigger those fitness adaptations, but remember the principle of progressive overload. Going from 15 miles (24.1km) a week to 30 miles (48.2km) a week in one fell swoop isn't progressive! Similarly, there's no point in following one that doesn't present a training stimulus because it's too easy (though bear in mind that the intensity is *meant* to be light during the Foundation phase, while you focus on building endurance).

Once you get started, keep a note on what you do and how you feel. (*See* 'Dear Diary' on p. 61.) If you find that it's too much – or not enough – you can always switch to a different plan.

# Understanding the plans

The runs are described in one of two ways. First, using terminology that I have explained in 'The jargon' on p. 62 (such as lactate threshold (LT) pace, tempo, steady run, easy run). The best way to remind yourself of what these runs should feel like, in terms of effort level, is to check the 'Monitoring Intensity table' on pp. 278–9. This table also gives heart rate and pace guidelines.

If the session involves repetitions (reps), the number of reps and sets is indicated, as well as the length of the recovery. The recovery may be a jog, or complete rest. For example, '3 x 9 mins LT pace with 2 mins jog' means run the 9 minutes three times, jogging for 2 minutes between each one.

The other method I use in the plans is ascribing a run (or sections of it) a particular pace, such as your '1-mile pace' or '10K pace'. This refers to your best recent pace over the stated distance. What if you have never timed or raced a mile, or have no idea what your 'best' 3K pace is? I recommend using a race prediction calculator, such as the McMillan

Running Pace Calculator, to get an estimated pace range (a few seconds either side of the 'prescribed' pace is absolutely fine) for any distance you don't know an approximate race pace for, using a recent race result as your baseline. Review this after any mid-training races. There are a few instances where the instructions may say '10K effort' instead of '10K pace'. This is because the session includes some hills, so trying to achieve the pace you would run on a flat surface isn't appropriate. It should feel like the same level of effort as running 10K on the flat, but the actual pace will fluctuate, along with the gradient.

A word about marathon pace (MP). Throughout the plans, I've included bouts within runs and entire runs at 'MP'. This assumes that MP is a step up from your easy running pace, which isn't always the case, especially for less fast runners. If you come across a run asking you to speed up to MP but doing so wouldn't make the run become any more challenging, increase your pace a little more (quicker than MP and maybe up to half-marathon pace, or HMP).

## Built-in flexibility

The sessions are presented on specific days. You can move them around if that fits better into your routine. However, try not to bunch hard runs and long runs too close together – ensure you have enough recovery between them. I've also suggested taking part in a race or Parkrun on certain days. Again, if you can't make those days, it's fine to miss them or move them around but do so with an awareness of the other sessions surrounding the 'race' day, as you may need to shift these, too.

I've indicated a dress rehearsal run on each plan. Again, this can be moved if necessary, but make sure you don't leave it too late, as you need to have the opportunity to adjust and retest anything within your strategy that doesn't work as well as you hoped.

You will notice that I use a mix of time (duration) and distance. There are two reasons for this. One is that the use of time enables quicker runners to accumulate more mileage. (For example, if the run is 40 minutes, someone whose 'easy' pace is around 8-minute-miling (4 mins 58 secs per km) will cover 5 miles (8km), while someone whose easy pace is around 10-minute-miling (6 mins 12 secs per km) will cover 4 miles (6.4km). If all the runs were prescribed by distance, slower runners would end up running for a much longer time overall than faster runners, and risk overtraining. However, we all need to run the same distance come race day – so it's important to include *some* distance-based runs in the plan, too. In some sessions, I offer a time or distance *range*, rather than a specific figure. Again, this is to allow the flexibility to do a little more or less, according to your capabilities and how you are feeling.

The second reason I mix time and distance is that it adds variety. When you're used to going out to run, say, 12 miles (19.3km) or 15 miles (24.1km), it can be quite refreshing to be asked to run for two hours, irrespective of distance – and it opens up the possibility of running on trails.

## The 'extras' – sprints, strides and surges

You will find that sprints, strides and surges feature in all the plans.

**Sprints** are all-out efforts. You are running as fast as you can for the (mercifully short) duration. Make sure you are well warmed up before you sprint and be wary of doing so when you are fatigued. If you are new to sprinting or feel nervous about it, hold back a little from a maximal effort.

**Strides** are short efforts – maybe 30m (33 yards) or 15–20 seconds – run at a fast pace, but not a sprint. You can perform them at the end of a warm-up or, Ethiopian style, at the end of a run. The focus is on running with good technique and staying relaxed. After you run a stride, walk back to your start point, to give you some recovery time before the next one. You should finish a set of strides feeling energised, not exhausted.

**Surges** are like strides, but they take place within a run. You pick up the pace (remember it's fast, but not a sprint) for the required duration and then return to the pace you were running at before. Try not to slow right down after the surge – the objective is to recover on the move. And transition into the surge, rather than exploding into it.

# DEAR DIARY - THE VIRTUES OF KEEPING NOTES

Maintaining a training journal is a great way of keeping your eye on the bigger picture of training. Research shows that people who do so are more consistent with their training than those who don't. Now, this probably reflects the fact that those who take the trouble to keep a journal are more invested in their training in the first place – but even so, there are lots of good reasons to follow suit.

1. It creates a record of what you did and what the results were, providing essential information for planning what to do next. (After all, there's little point in doing more of the same if it's not taking you in the right direction.) By 'results', I don't only mean race times but how your body responded to different sessions – how it felt at the time, how long it took you to recover, for example.

2. Regular reviews of what you've written allow patterns to be identified. Always exhausted on Thursdays? Perhaps you need to tweak your schedule to get more recovery after the Wednesday session. Feel fantastic two days after a sports massage? Schedule one in on the appropriate day before your next big race.

3. It's a great motivator. Flicking back a few pages (or reviewing your history, if you're using Strava or similar) shows you just how far you've come, spurring you on to keep making the effort. Or conversely, it can be the wake-up call you need if you've fallen off the programme.

4. Less positive, but no less useful, is the journal's function as a trail of clues if things go wrong. An injury that stops you in your tracks can often be traced back to a too-steep increase – or simply a sudden change – in training. Or perhaps external factors played a part, such as poor nutrition, too many late nights or long hours hunched at your desk – that's why recording as much information as possible in your training log is useful. A single word – 'stressed', 'hungover' – can speak volumes!

A training diary can be whatever you want it to be. It can be online or on paper. You could simply record how long, or how far, you ran and at what pace, or you could include how you felt on the run, what route you took, what the weather was like and what kind of mood you were in. It may take a little perseverance to make it a habit, but eventually it will become as much a part of your routine as running itself.

# THE JARGON

## Abbreviations

LT – lactate threshold

HMP – half-marathon pace

MP – marathon pace

Hrs – hours

Mins – minutes

Secs – seconds

X/x – times, as in the number of times to do something

## Pace/effort descriptions included

1-mile pace – based on a prediction from a recent race.

3K pace – based on a prediction from a recent race.

5K pace – based on a prediction from a recent race.

10K pace – based on a prediction from a recent race.

LT pace – if your 10K time is an hour or more, then your LT pace will be the same or a little faster than 10K pace. The more below an hour your 10K pace is, the slower your LT pace will be in comparison – typically 5–15 seconds slower per mile.

Tempo pace – this will be just a few seconds per mile slower than your LT pace. E.g. 3–5 secs.

Steady pace – based on feel.

HMP – based on a prediction from a recent race.

MP – based on your marathon goal time.

Easy – based on feel.

Very easy – based on feel.

## Other terminology

Reps – repetitions; the number of times to run the time or distance specified.

Sets – a 'group' of repetitions. You may be asked to do more than one set of reps, with a recovery jog or rest between them.

Progression run – a run that gradually increases in pace as time progresses.

Fast finish – an easy run that finishes at a faster pace.

## Hill choice

The hill you use for the hill sprints should be steep (7%-plus gradient). But you need to be able to run with good posture and technique. If you can't, choose a shallower slope.

For the more traditional hill reps in the programmes, the gradient should be moderately steep, around 5–6%.

For hilly circuits/runs, it's not important as long as there are some climbs and descents of various lengths and gradients.

# The Full Throttle plans (see pp. 66-73)

The Full Throttle Experienced programme mostly involves training five days per week, with a sprinkling of six-day weeks. Since it is presented in a mix of miles and minutes, it's not possible to give an exact weekly mileage. However, to give a ballpark figure and point of comparison with the other programmes, a runner averaging 10-minute miles (6 mins 12 secs per km) across all sessions would average 30 miles (48.3km) a week overall (excluding taper), peaking at around 37 miles (59.5km). The Full Throttle First-timer programme begins with four days a week, building to five after the first few weeks. I estimate runners will average 26 miles (41.8km) a week overall, peaking at around 33 miles (53.1km).

- You'll notice I haven't followed the classic 'speedwork on Tuesdays, tempo on Thursdays' approach. I prefer to place the week's main 'quality' session on a Wednesday (giving one full rest day and one easy day after the long run). Adding in a low volume of additional high-intensity training on a Saturday works because, despite not following the 'hard-easy' rule, the amount isn't high enough to fatigue you for your long run – (apart from when it's actually meant to!)
- Some flexibility is offered on the Tuesday run (Experienced level plan only) by giving a fairly broad time range (e.g. 45–60 minutes) and on Wednesday workouts by giving a suggested range of reps, rather than a concrete number. Don't automatically go for the higher end of the suggested duration range or the greatest number of repeats (or the lowest, for that matter!). Consider what is most appropriate for you, based on your fitness, your aspirations and on the amount of training you were doing leading up to starting the plan. Remember, we don't want any sudden leaps in mileage.

# The Steady State plans (see pp. 74-81)

These Steady State plans are lower in volume than the Full Throttle ones, but many of the sessions are similar. At both levels, the programmes are mostly four days per week, with a handful of five-day weeks.

- Some of the easy runs are longer than on the Full Throttle plans, because there are fewer in total and this helps to maintain volume. The programmes mix distance (miles) with time (minutes) so the total weekly mileage will differ from person to person. A runner averaging 10-minute miles (6 mins 12 secs per km) across all training sessions would cover 27 miles (43.5km) a week overall (excluding taper) and peak at around 34 miles (54.7km) in the Experienced plan and 26 miles (41.8km) a week in the First-timer plan, peaking at 32 miles (51.5km).
- As with the Full Throttle plans, the week's main 'quality' session (hills or speedwork) is on a Wednesday (giving one full rest day and one easy day after the long run). Some flexibility is offered on the Tuesday run (from the beginning on the Experienced level plan and after the Foundation phase on the First-timer plan) by giving a fairly broad time range (e.g. 30–45 minutes) and on Wednesday sessions by giving a suggested range of reps, rather than a set figure. Choose what is most appropriate for you, based on your fitness, your aspirations and on the amount of training you were doing leading up to starting the plan.

# The Minimalist plans (see pp. 82-89)

My Minimalist plans are the lowest-volume option. They are designed for people who are short on time for running, or who want to restrict the amount of running they do in marathon training for another reason, such as concerns about injury. At both levels, training is mostly three days a week, with a few four-day weeks within the Specific phase and to accommodate races or Parkruns. The 'quality' workouts shift to a

Thursday on these plans, to space three days of training out more evenly through the week. The volume of these workouts is a little lower than on the other plans to avoid an imbalance, though weekday easy runs are sometimes longer than on the other plans to boost volume.

- The long runs are slightly fewer and on the First-timer plan, they are given as either a distance or time goal. Depending on individual pace, some runners may not reach 20 miles (32km) on their peak long run. (Don't be alarmed about this – the Hanson brothers' marathon-training programmes never go beyond 16 miles/25.7km for long runs – and I ran my first marathon successfully having never covered more than 18 miles/29km).
- On these Minimalist plans, a runner averaging 10-minute-miling (6 mins 12 secs per km) across all training runs would be running approximately 25 miles (40.2km) a week overall in the Experienced level plan, peaking at around 30 miles (48.3km). The same runner following the First-timer plan would average 23 miles (37km) a week overall, peaking at 30 miles (48.3km) or five hours of running.

| Week | Phase | Monday | Tuesday | Wednesday | |
|------|-------|--------|---------|-----------|--|
| 1 | Foundation | Rest | 30–45 mins easy | 40 mins easy plus 4–6 x 15-sec strides | |
| 2 | Foundation | Rest | 35–50 mins easy | 45 mins easy with surges of 30 secs every 5th minute (9 in total) | |
| 3 | Foundation | Rest | 35–50 mins easy | 10 mins easy, then alternate 45 secs easy/45 secs hard (1-mile–3K pace) x 5. Jog 5 mins. Repeat the 45-sec reps | |
| 4 | Foundation | Rest | 35–50 mins easy | 15 mins easy, then run 45, 90, 45 secs hard (3–5K pace) with 60-sec jogs between each effort x 3 sets. Jog 3 mins between sets | |
| 5 | Foundation | Rest | 35–50 mins easy | 45 mins easy including 6–8 x 45–60-sec hill reps at 5K effort, with untimed recoveries | |
| 6 | Foundation | Rest | 40–55 mins easy | 15 mins easy, then 5–6 x 2 mins at 5K pace with 2-min jogs between reps | |
| 7 | Development | Rest | 40–55 mins easy | 15 mins easy, then 25 mins on a hilly route or circuit, pushing to 10K effort on the climbs, recovering on the flats. Or 15 mins easy then 3–5 long hill repeats (2–3 mins each) on a shallow hill at 10K effort, recovering at a jog, no rest | |
| 8 | Development | 30 mins very easy or rest | 35–50 mins easy | 15 mins easy, then 4–5 x 3 mins at 5K pace with 2-min jogs between reps. Or do Saturday's session if doing Parkrun on Saturday | |
| 9 | Development | Rest | 45–60 mins easy | 10 mins easy, 25 mins tempo, 10 mins steady | |
| 10 | Development | 30 mins very easy or rest | 30–45 mins easy | 15 mins easy, then 4 x 7–8 mins at LT pace, with a surge on the last minute of each rep and 90 secs rest between reps | |

| Thursday | Friday | Saturday | Sunday |
|---|---|---|---|
| 40 mins easy | Rest | 30 mins easy plus 4 x 10-sec hill sprints | Long run 13 miles (20.9km) easy |
| 40 mins easy | Rest | 30 mins easy plus 5 x 10-sec hill sprints | Long run 14 miles (22.5km) easy |
| 40 mins easy | Rest | 30 mins easy plus 6 x 10-sec hill sprints | Mid-long run 9–10 miles (14.5–16km) easy or 90 mins trail |
| 40 mins easy | Rest | 40 mins easy plus 6 x 10-sec hill sprints | Long run with fast finish. 15 miles (24km), picking up pace over last 10–15 mins |
| 30 mins very easy | Rest | 40 mins easy plus 4 x 20-sec flat sprints | Long run 16 miles (25.7km) easy |
| 40 mins easy | Rest | 10 mins easy, 20 mins tempo | 6 miles (9.7km) steady |
| 40 mins easy | Rest | 40 mins easy plus 4 x 20-sec flat sprints | Long run 18 miles (29km) easy |
| 40 mins easy | Rest | 40 mins easy plus 6 x 10-sec hill sprints or Parkrun | Mid-long run 10 miles (16km), picking up to MP or a little quicker over final 4 miles (6.4km). Or a 10-mile (16km) race (not in addition to Parkrun) |
| 30 mins very easy | Rest | 40 mins easy | Long run 20 miles (32km) easy or equivalent in predicted duration on trail. No longer than 3 hrs 30 mins |
| 40 mins steady | Rest | 45 mins easy including 6–8 x 45–60-sec hill reps at 5K effort, with untimed recoveries | 5 miles (8km) with last 20 mins at goal HMP |

# Full Throttle Plan | Experienced ▸ Weeks 11–20

| Week | Phase | Monday | Tuesday | Wednesday | |
|------|-------|--------|---------|-----------|---|
| 11 | Development | Rest | 35–50 mins steady | 10 mins easy, 25 mins tempo, 10 mins steady. Or if not racing, do Wednesday session from week 7 | |
| 12 | Development | Rest | 30–45 mins very easy | 15 mins easy, then 'Unders and Overs': alternate 60 secs at LT pace with 30 secs a little faster for 4 reps (6 mins in total per rep) x 3 sets, 2 mins 30 secs rest between sets | |
| 13 | Specific | Rest | 30–45 mins very easy or rest | 15 mins easy, then 3 x 9–10 mins at LT pace with 2 mins jogging between reps | |
| 14 | Specific | 30 mins very easy | 35–50 mins steady | 15 mins easy then 'Mile Winders': 1st mile at approx. MP, then each subsequent mile a few secs (3–10 secs) quicker. Aim for 4–5 reps with 90 secs rest between reps | |
| 15 | Specific | 40 mins steady | 45–60 mins easy | 15 mins easy, then 15 mins tempo, 2 mins easy, 10 mins at 10K pace, 2 mins easy, 5 mins at 5K pace, 2 mins easy, 2 mins at 1-mile–3K pace | |
| 16 | Specific | Rest | 30–45 mins very easy or rest | 10 mins easy then alternating 2 mins at MP, 1 min at LT pace for 9 mins. Jog for 5 mins and repeat x 2 more sets | |
| 17 | Specific | Rest | 30–45 mins very easy or rest | 10 mins easy, 25–30 mins tempo, 2 mins rest, then 5 x 60 secs at 1-mile–3K pace with 60 secs rest between reps | |
| 18 | Taper | Rest | 30–40 mins easy | 10 mins easy, then 5 mins LT pace, 2 mins easy, 5 mins LT pace, 2 mins easy, 2 mins 5K pace, 5 mins easy | |
| 19 | Taper | Rest | 20–40 mins very easy | 5 miles (8km) steady with surge to MP or HMP for 1 min at the end of each 1 mile (1.6km) | |
| 20 | Taper | Rest | 20–40 mins easy with 3 x 15-sec strides | 4 miles (6.4km) easy with last 1 mile (1.6km) at MP or a little faster | |

| Thursday | Friday | Saturday | Sunday |
|---|---|---|---|
| 30 mins very easy | Rest | 30 mins easy plus 3–5 x 15-sec strides | Half-marathon race |
| 40 mins easy | Rest | 40 mins steady | Long run 20 miles (32km) easy. No longer than 3 hrs 30 mins |
| 40 mins easy | Rest | 40 mins easy plus 6 x 10-sec hill sprints | 2-hr long run with progression: 30 mins easy, 30 mins MP, 10 mins easy, 10 mins MP, 10 mins easy, 10 mins HMP, 10 mins LT, 10 mins easy |
| 40 mins easy | Rest | 6 miles (9.7km) at MP plus 3–5 x 15-sec strides or Parkrun | 9–10 miles (14.5–16km) easy or 80–90 mins on trail |
| 40 mins easy | Rest | 30 mins very easy | 3 miles (4.8km) easy then 4 x 15 mins at MP with 1 mile (1.6km) easy between each block, then 2 miles (3.2km) easy DRESS REHEARSAL |
| 30 mins easy | Rest | 40 mins steady plus 3–5 15-sec strides | Long run 20 miles (32km) easy. No longer than 3 hrs 30 mins |
| 40 mins easy | Rest | 40 mins steady | 3 miles (4.8km) easy, then 3 x 20 mins at MP with 1 mile (1.6km) easy between each block, then 2 miles (3.2km) easy |
| 20–30 mins very easy | Rest | 40 mins easy plus 3–5 x 15-sec strides | 30 mins easy, 30 mins MP, 30 mins easy |
| 20–30 mins very easy | Rest | 30 mins easy plus 3 x 15-sec strides | 30 mins easy, 30 mins MP |
| 20–30 mins very easy or rest | Rest | 20–30 mins easy or rest | Race day |

# Full Throttle Plan | First-timer ▶ Weeks 1–10

| Week | Phase | Monday | Tuesday | Wednesday | |
|------|-------|--------|---------|-----------|---|
| 1 | Foundation | Rest | 30 mins easy | 40 mins easy plus 4–6 x 15-sec strides | |
| 2 | Foundation | Rest | 30 mins easy | 40 mins easy with surges of 30 secs every 5th minute | |
| 3 | Foundation | Rest | 35 mins easy | 10 mins easy, then alternate 30 secs easy/30 secs hard (approx. 3K pace) x 5. Jog 5 mins. Repeat the 30-sec reps | |
| 4 | Foundation | Rest | 35 mins easy | 15 mins easy, then 45, 90, 45 secs hard (3–5K pace) with 60 secs rest between efforts x 2 sets. Jog 5 mins between sets | |
| 5 | Foundation | Rest | 35 mins easy | 45 mins easy including 6–8 x 30–45-sec hill reps at 5K effort on moderate hill, with untimed recoveries. Then 10 mins tempo | |
| 6 | Foundation | Rest | 40 mins easy | 15 mins easy, then 5 x 1 min at 3–5K pace with 1 min rest between. Jog 5 mins and repeat. If doing Parkrun, do Saturday's session instead | |
| 7 | Foundation | Rest | 40 mins easy | 15 mins easy, then 20 mins on a hilly route or circuit, pushing to 10K effort on the climbs, recovering on the flats. Or 15 mins easy then 3–5 long hill repeats (90–120 secs each) on a shallow hill at 10K effort, recovering at a jog, no rest | |
| 8 | Foundation | Rest | 40 mins easy | 15 mins easy, then 3 x 2 mins at 5K pace with 2 mins rest between. Jog 5 mins then repeat the set. 15 mins easy | |
| 9 | Development | Rest | 40–50 mins easy | 10 mins easy, 20 mins tempo, 10 mins steady | |
| 10 | Development | Rest | 40–50 mins easy | 15 mins easy, then 4 x 6–7 mins at LT pace with 90 secs slow jog between reps | |

| Thursday | Friday | Saturday | Sunday |
|----------|--------|----------|--------|
| Rest | 30 mins easy plus 4 x 10-sec hill sprints | Rest | Long run 12 miles (19.3km) easy |
| Rest | 30 mins easy plus 5 x 10-sec hill sprints | Rest | Long run 13 miles (20.9km) easy |
| Rest | 30 mins easy plus 6 x 10-sec hill sprints | Rest | Mid-long run 8–9 miles (12.9–14.5km) easy |
| Rest | 40 mins easy plus 6 x 10-sec hill sprints | Rest | Long run 14 miles (22.5km) easy or add 10 mins to duration it took to run 13 miles (20.9km) in week 2 and run equivalent duration on trail (do NOT worry about distance covered) |
| Rest | 40 mins easy plus 4 x 20-sec flat sprints | Rest | Long run 15 miles (24km), speeding up a little over final 10–15 mins |
| Rest | 40 mins easy | Parkrun or 5 miles (8km) steady plus 4 x 20-sec flat sprints | 30 mins very easy |
| Rest | 45 mins easy | Rest | Long run 16 miles (25.7km) easy |
| Rest | 20 mins easy, 10 mins tempo plus 6 x 10-sec hill sprints | Rest | Long run 18 miles (29km). No longer than 3 hrs 15 mins |
| 30 mins very easy | Rest | 40 mins steady | Mid-long run 10 miles (16km); start easy and pick up to MP or a little quicker over final 4 miles (6.4km) |
| Rest | 40 mins easy plus 3–5 x 15-sec strides | Rest | Long run 20 miles (32km) or equivalent in predicted duration on trail. No longer than 3 hrs 30 mins |

# Full Throttle Plan | First-timer ▸ Weeks 11–20

| Week | Phase | Monday | Tuesday | Wednesday | |
|------|-------|--------|---------|-----------|---|
| 11 | Development | Rest | 30 mins very easy | 15 mins easy, then 'Unders and Overs': alternate 60 secs at LT pace with 30 secs a little faster for 4 sets (6 mins in total per set) x 3 sets, 2 mins 30 secs rest between sets | |
| 12 | Development | Rest | 40–50 mins easy | 10 mins easy, 25 mins tempo, 5 mins easy | |
| 13 | Specific | Rest | 30 mins easy plus 4 x 10-sec hill sprints | 15 mins easy, then 3 x 8–9 mins at LT pace with 2 mins slow jog between reps | |
| 14 | Specific | Rest | 40–50 mins easy | 10 mins easy then alternating 2 mins MP, 1 min LT pace for 9 mins. Jog for 5 mins and repeat | |
| 15 | Specific | Rest | 30–40 mins easy | 5–7 miles (8–11.3km) progression run: start easy, pick up to MP and last 2 miles (3.2km) HMP | |
| 16 | Specific | Rest | 30–40 mins easy | 15 mins easy then 'Mile Winders': 1st mile at approx. MP, then each subsequent 1 mile (1.6km) a few secs (3–10 secs) quicker. Aim for 4 reps with 90 secs rest between reps | |
| 17 | Specific | Rest | 40–50 mins easy | 10 mins easy, 20–25 mins tempo, 2 mins rest, then 5 x 45 secs at 1-mile–3K pace with 45 secs rest between reps | |
| 18 | Taper | Rest | 40–50 mins easy | 10 mins easy, then 5 mins LT pace, 2 mins easy, 5 mins LT pace, 2 mins easy, 2 mins 5K pace, 5 mins easy | |
| 19 | Taper | Rest | 20–30 mins very easy | 5 miles (8km) steady with surge to MP or HMP for 1 min at the end of each 1 mile (1.6km) | |
| 20 | Taper | Rest | 20–30 mins easy with 3 x 15-sec strides | 4 miles (6.4km) easy with last 1 mile (1.6km) at MP or a little faster | |

| Thursday | Friday | Saturday | Sunday |
|---|---|---|---|
| 40–50 mins easy | Rest | 45 mins easy including 6–8 x 30–45-sec hill reps at 5K effort, with untimed recoveries | 60 mins steady |
| 30 mins very easy | Rest | 25 mins easy plus 3 x 15-sec strides | Half-marathon race |
| 30 mins very easy | Rest | 30 mins very easy | Long run 20 miles (32km). No longer than 3 hrs 30 mins DRESS REHEARSAL |
| 30 mins very easy | Rest | 7 miles (11.3km) easy | 3 miles (4.8km) then 3 x 15 mins at MP with 1 mile (1.6km) easy between each block, then 3 miles (4.8km) easy |
| 40 mins easy | Rest | 15 mins easy, then 4 x 4 mins each run as 3 mins 10K pace, 1 min 5K pace with 2-min rest between reps. 15 mins easy. Or Parkrun | 60 mins steady |
| 30 mins steady | Rest | 30 mins easy plus 3 x 15-sec strides | Long run 18 miles (29km) – first half easy, second half steady. No longer than 3 hrs DRESS REHEARSAL |
| 30 mins very easy | Rest | 6 miles (9.7km) easy | 2-hr run with progression: 30 mins easy, 30 mins MP, 15 mins easy, 15 mins MP, 10 mins easy, 10 mins HMP, 10 mins easy |
| 40 mins easy | Rest | 30 mins steady | 20 mins easy, 30 mins MP, 10 mins HMP, 20 mins easy |
| 30 mins easy plus 3 x 15-sec strides | Rest | 30 mins steady | 30 mins easy, 20 mins MP |
| Rest | 20–30 mins easy or rest | Rest | Race day |

## Steady State | Experienced ▸ Weeks 1–10

| Week | Phase | Monday | Tuesday | Wednesday | |
|------|-------|--------|---------|-----------|---|
| 1 | Foundation | Rest | 35–50 mins easy | 40 mins easy plus 4–6 x 15-sec strides | |
| 2 | Foundation | Rest | 35–50 mins easy | 10 mins easy, then alternate 45 secs easy/45 secs at 1-mile–3K pace x 5. Jog 5 mins. Repeat the 45-sec reps | |
| 3 | Foundation | Rest | 35–50 mins easy | 50 mins easy with surges of 30 secs every 5th minute (10 in total) | |
| 4 | Foundation | Rest | 35–50 mins easy | 15 mins easy. 45, 90, 45 secs at 3–5K pace, with 60 secs rest between each x 3 sets. Jog 3 mins between sets | |
| 5 | Foundation | Rest | 35–50 mins easy | 45 mins easy, including 6–8 x 45–60-sec hill reps at 5K effort, with untimed recoveries, then 10 mins tempo | |
| 6 | Foundation | Rest | 40–55 mins easy | 15 mins easy, then 5–6 x 2 mins at 5K pace, with 2 mins easy jog between reps | |
| 7 | Development | Rest | 40–55 mins easy | 10 mins easy, 20 mins tempo, 10 mins steady | |
| 8 | Development | Rest | 40–55 mins easy | 15 mins easy, then 25 mins on a hilly route or circuit, pushing to 10K effort on the climbs, recovering on the flats. Or 15 mins easy then 3–5 long hill repeats (2–3 mins each) on a shallow hill at 10K effort, recovering at a jog, no rest. If doing Parkrun on Saturday, do Saturday's run instead | |
| 9 | Development | Rest | 45–60 mins easy | 10 mins easy, 25 mins tempo, 10 mins steady | |
| 10 | Development | Rest | 30–45 mins very easy | 15 mins easy, then 4 x 6–7 mins at LT pace, with 90 secs rest between reps. Surge to faster pace for last 1 min of each rep | |

| Thursday | Friday | Saturday | Sunday |
|---|---|---|---|
| Rest | 30 mins easy plus 4 x 10-sec hill sprints | Rest | Long run 13 miles (20.9km) easy |
| Rest | 30 mins easy plus 5 x 10-sec hill sprints | Rest | Mid-long run 9–10 miles (14.5–16km) easy or 75–90 mins trail |
| Rest | 40 mins easy plus 6 x 10-sec hill sprints | Rest | Long run 14 miles (22.5km) easy |
| Rest | 40 mins easy plus 6 x 10-sec hill sprints | Rest | Long run with fast finish. 15 miles (24km), picking up pace over last 10–15 mins |
| Rest | 40 mins easy plus 4 x 20-sec flat sprints | Rest | 7 miles (11.3km) steady |
| Rest | 40 mins steady | Rest | Long run 16 miles (25.7km) easy |
| Rest | 50 mins easy | Rest | Long run 18 miles (29km) easy |
| 30 mins very easy | Rest | 40 mins easy plus 4 x 20-sec flat sprints, or Parkrun | Mid-long run 10 miles (16km), picking up to MP or a little quicker over final 4 miles (6.4km). Or a 10-mile (16km) race (not in addition to Parkrun) |
| Rest | 50 mins easy plus 3 x 15-sec strides | Rest | Long run 20 miles (32km) easy or equivalent in predicted duration on trail. Duration no longer than 3 hrs 30 mins |
| 40 mins easy | Rest | 45 mins easy, including 6–8 x 45–60-sec hill reps at 5K effort, with untimed recoveries | 60 mins easy |

# Steady State | Experienced ▸ Weeks 11–20

| Week | Phase | Monday | Tuesday | Wednesday | |
|------|-------|--------|---------|-----------|---|
| 11 | Development | Rest | 15 mins easy, then 3 x 9–10 mins at LT pace with 2 mins rest | 35–50 mins steady | |
| 12 | Development | Rest | 30–45 mins very easy or rest | 15 mins easy, then 'Unders and Overs': alternate 60 secs just below LT pace with 30 secs a little faster for 4 reps (6 mins in total per rep) x 3 sets, with 2 mins 30 secs rest between sets | |
| 13 | Specific | Rest | 30–45 mins very easy | 5–7-mile (8–11.3km) progression run: start easy, pick up to MP and last 2 miles (3.2km) HMP | |
| 14 | Specific | Rest | 35–50 mins steady | 15 mins easy, 30 mins tempo | |
| 15 | Specific | Rest | 35–50 mins easy | 10 mins easy then alternating 2 mins MP, 1 min at LT pace for 9 mins. Jog for 5 mins and repeat x 2 more sets | |
| 16 | Specific | Rest | 30–45 mins very easy or rest | 15 mins easy then 'Mile Winders': 1st mile at approx. MP, then each subsequent mile 3–10 secs quicker. Aim for 4–5 reps, with 90 secs rest between reps | |
| 17 | Specific | Rest | 35–50 mins easy | 10 mins easy, 25–30 mins tempo, 2 mins rest, then 5 x 60 secs at 1-mile–3km pace, with 60 secs rest between reps | |
| 18 | Taper | Rest | 50 mins easy | 10 mins easy, then 5 mins LT pace, 2 mins easy, 5 mins LT pace, 2 mins easy, 2 mins at 5K pace, 5 mins easy | |
| 19 | Taper | Rest | 30–40 mins very easy | 5 miles (8km) steady, with surge to MP or HMP for 1 min at the end of each 1 mile (1.6km) | |
| 20 | Taper | Rest | 20–40 mins easy with 3 x 15-sec strides | 4 miles (6.4km) easy, with last 1 mile (1.6km) MP or a little faster | |

| Thursday | Friday | Saturday | Sunday |
|---|---|---|---|
| 40 mins easy | Rest | 30 mins easy plus 3–5 x 15-sec strides | Half-marathon race |
| Rest | 30 mins steady | Rest | Long run 20 miles (32km) easy. Duration no longer than 3 hrs 30 mins |
| Rest | 40 mins easy plus 6 x 10-sec hill sprints | Rest | 10 miles (16km) easy, or 80–90 mins on trail, or rest |
| Rest | 50 mins easy | 30 mins very easy | 3 miles (4.8km) easy then 4 x 15 mins MP with 1 mile (1.6km) easy between each block, then 2 miles (3.2km) easy |
| Rest | 40 mins steady | Rest | Long run 20 miles (32km) easy. Aim to run 2nd half a little faster than first half by starting out easy. Duration no longer than 3hrs 30 mins. DRESS REHEARSAL |
| 40 mins easy | Rest | 40–50 mins MP plus 3–5 x 15-sec strides, or Parkrun | 10 miles (16km) easy or 80–90 mins on trail |
| 30 mins very easy | Rest | 7–8 miles (11.3–12.9km) easy | 2-hr long run with progression: 30 mins easy, 30 mins MP, 15 mins easy, 15 mins MP, 10 mins easy, 10 mins HMP, 10 mins LT, 10 mins easy |
| Rest | 5–6 miles (8–9.7km) easy | Rest | 30 mins easy, 30 mins MP, 30 mins easy |
| Rest | 30 mins easy plus 3 x 15-sec strides | Rest | 30 mins easy, 30 mins MP |
| Rest | 20–30 mins easy or rest | Rest | Race day |

# Steady State | First-timer ▸ Weeks 1–10

| Week | Phase | Monday | Tuesday | Wednesday | |
|------|-------|--------|---------|-----------|---|
| 1 | Foundation | Rest | 30 mins easy | 40 mins easy plus 4–6 x 15-sec strides | |
| 2 | Foundation | Rest | 30 mins easy | 10 mins easy, then alternate 30 secs easy/30 secs hard (approx 3K pace) x 5. Jog 5 mins. Repeat the 30-sec reps | |
| 3 | Foundation | Rest | 35 mins easy | 40 mins easy with surges of 30 secs every 5th minute (8 in total) | |
| 4 | Foundation | Rest | 35 mins easy | 15 mins easy, then 45, 90, 45 secs hard (3–5K pace) with 60 secs rest between efforts x 2 sets. Jog 5 mins between sets | |
| 5 | Foundation | Rest | 40 mins easy | 45 mins easy, including 6–8 x 30–45-sec hill reps at 5K effort on moderate hill, with untimed recoveries | |
| 6 | Foundation | Rest | 40 mins easy | 15 mins easy, then 5 x 1 min at 3–5K pace with 1-min rest between reps. Jog 5 mins and repeat | |
| 7 | Foundation | Rest | 45 mins easy | 10 mins easy, 10 mins tempo, 2 mins jog, then 3 x 2 mins at 3–5K pace, with 2 mins rest between reps | |
| 8 | Foundation | Rest | 45 mins easy | 15 mins easy, then 20 mins on a hilly route or circuit, pushing to 10K effort on the climbs, recovering on the flats. Or 15 mins easy then 3–5 long hill repeats (90–120 secs each) on a shallow hill at 10K effort, recovering at a jog, no rest | |
| 9 | Development | Rest | 45–60 mins easy | 10 mins easy, 20 mins tempo, 10 mins steady | |
| 10 | Development | Rest or cross-train | 30–45 mins very easy | 15 mins easy, then 4 x 6–7 mins at LT pace, with 90 secs rest between reps. Surge to faster pace for last 30 secs of each rep | |

| Thursday | Friday | Saturday | Sunday |
|---|---|---|---|
| Rest | 30 mins easy plus 4 x 10-sec hill sprints | Rest or cross-train | Long run 12 miles (19.3km) easy |
| Rest | 30 mins easy plus 5 x 10-sec hill sprints | Rest or cross-train | Mid-long run 8–9 miles (12.9–14.5km) easy or 75–90 mins trail |
| Rest | 40 mins easy plus 6 x 10-sec hill sprints | Rest or cross-train | Long run 13 miles (20.9km) easy |
| Rest | 40 mins easy plus 6 x 10-sec hill sprints | Rest or cross-train | Long run 15 miles (24km) easy |
| Rest | Rest | Parkrun or 4 miles (6.4km) steady plus 4 x 20-sec flat sprints | 7 miles (11.3km) easy |
| Rest | 50 mins easy | Rest or cross-train | Long run 16 miles (25.7km), picking up pace over last 10–15 mins |
| Rest | 40 mins easy | Rest or cross-train | Long run 18 miles (29km) easy |
| Rest | 40 mins easy plus 4 x 20-sec flat sprints | Rest or cross-train | 60 mins easy |
| Rest | 30 mins easy plus 3 x 15-sec strides | Rest | Half-marathon race |
| Rest | 40 mins easy plus 3-5 x 15-sec strides | Rest | Long run 19–20 miles (30.6–32km) or equivalent in predicted duration on trail. Duration no longer than 3 hrs 20 mins |

## Steady State | First-timer ▸ Weeks 11–20

| Week | Phase | Monday | Tuesday | Wednesday | |
|------|-------|--------|---------|-----------|---|
| 11 | Development | Rest | 30–45 mins very easy or rest | 15 mins easy, then 3 x 8–9 mins at LT pace, with 2 mins rest between reps | |
| 12 | Development | Rest or cross-train | 45–60 mins easy | 15 mins easy, then 4 x 4 mins, each run as 3 mins 10K pace, 1 min 5K pace, with 2-min rest between reps | |
| 13 | Specific | Rest | 30–45 mins very easy | 5–7-mile (8–11.3km) progression run: start easy, pick up to MP and last 2 miles (3.2km) HMP | |
| 14 | Specific | Rest | 35–50 mins steady | 15 mins easy, 25–30 mins tempo | |
| 15 | Specific | Rest | 35–50 mins easy | 10 mins easy then alternating 2 mins MP, 1 min LT pace for 6 mins. Jog for 5 mins and repeat x 2 more sets | |
| 16 | Specific | Rest | 30–45 mins very easy or rest | 15 mins easy then 'Mile Winders': 1st mile at approx. MP, then each subsequent mile 3–10 secs quicker. Aim for 4–5 reps with 90 secs rest between reps | |
| 17 | Specific | Rest | 40–50 mins easy | 10 mins easy, 20–25 mins tempo, 2 mins rest, then 5 x 45 secs at 1-mile–3K pace, with 45 secs rest between reps | |
| 18 | Taper | Rest | 40 mins easy | 10 mins easy, then 5 mins LT pace, 2 mins easy, 5 mins LT pace, 2 mins easy, 2 mins 5K pace, 5 mins easy | |
| 19 | Taper | Rest | 30–40 mins very easy | 4 miles (6.4km) steady, with surge to MP or HMP for 1 min at the end of each 1 mile (1.6km) | |
| 20 | Taper | Rest | 20–30 mins easy with 3 x 15-sec strides | 4 miles (6.4km), 3 miles (4.8km) easy, with last mile MP or a little faster | |

| Thursday | Friday | Saturday | Sunday |
|---|---|---|---|
| Rest | 45 mins easy, including 6–8 x 30–45-sec hill reps at 5K effort, with untimed recoveries | Rest or cross-train | Mid-long run 8–9 miles (12.9–14.5km) easy or 75–90 mins trail |
| Rest | 30 mins steady | Rest | Long run 20 miles (32km). Duration no longer than 3 hrs 30 mins |
| Rest | 40 mins easy plus 6 x 10-sec hill sprints | Rest | 10 miles (16km) easy, or 90–100 mins on trail, or rest |
| 50 mins easy | Rest | 30 mins very easy | 3 miles (4.8km) then 3–4 x 15 mins MP with 1 mile (1.6km) easy between each block, then 2 miles (3.2km) easy |
| Rest | 40 mins steady | Rest | Long run 20 miles (32km) easy. Duration no longer than 3 hrs 30 mins. DRESS REHEARSAL |
| 40 mins easy | Rest | 30–40 mins steady plus 3 x 15-sec strides, or Parkrun | 9 miles (14.5km) easy or 80–90 mins on trail |
| Rest | 6–7 miles (9.7–11.3km) easy | Rest | 2-hr progression run: 30 mins easy, 30 mins MP, 15 mins easy, 15 mins MP, 10 mins easy, 10 mins HMP, 10 mins easy |
| Rest | 4–5 miles (6.4–8km) easy | Rest | 90 mins easy |
| Rest | 30 mins easy plus 3 x 15-sec strides | Rest | 30 mins easy, 20 mins MP |
| Rest | 20–30 mins easy or rest | Rest | Race day |

| Week | Phase | Monday | Tuesday | Wednesday | |
|------|-------|--------|---------|-----------|---|
| 1 | Foundation | Rest | 40 mins easy plus 4 x 10-sec hill sprints | Rest | |
| 2 | Foundation | Rest | 40 mins easy plus 5 x 10-sec hill sprints | Rest | |
| 3 | Foundation | Rest | 45 mins easy plus 6 x 10-sec hill sprints | Rest | |
| 4 | Foundation | Rest | 45 mins easy plus 6 x 10-sec hill sprints | Rest | |
| 5 | Foundation | Rest | 45 mins easy plus 4 x 20-sec flat sprints | Rest | |
| 6 | Foundation | Rest | 45 mins easy plus 6 x 10-sec hill sprints | Rest | |
| 7 | Development | Rest | 40 mins steady | Rest | |
| 8 | Development | Rest | 50 mins easy plus 4 x 20-sec flat sprints | Rest | |
| 9 | Development | Rest | 50 mins easy | Rest | |
| 10 | Development | Rest | 50 mins easy plus 4 x 10-sec hill sprints or 3 x 20-sec flat sprints | Rest | |

| Thursday | Friday | Saturday | Sunday |
|---|---|---|---|
| 40 mins easy with surges of 30 secs every 5th minute (8 in total) | Rest or cross-train | Rest | Long run 12 miles (19.3km) easy |
| 15 mins easy, then alternate 45 secs easy/45 secs 1-mile–3K pace x 6. 15 mins easy | Rest or cross-train | Rest | Long run 13 miles (20.9km) easy |
| 15 mins easy, then 8 x 1 min at 3–5K pace, with 1-min rest between reps. Jog 5 mins, then 10 mins tempo. If doing Parkrun, do Saturday's session instead | Rest or cross-train | Parkrun or 30 mins steady | Mid-long run 10 miles (16km) easy or 90 mins trail |
| 60 mins easy | Rest or cross-train | Rest | Long run with fast finish. 14 miles (22.5km), picking up pace over last 10–15 mins |
| 45 mins easy including 6–8 x 45–60 sec hill reps at 5K effort, with untimed recoveries then 10 mins tempo | Rest or cross-train | 8 miles (12.9km) easy | 7 miles (11.3km) steady |
| 15 mins easy, then 4 x 2 mins at 5K pace with 2 mins easy jog between reps, then 10 mins tempo | Rest or cross-train | Rest | Long run 16 miles (25.7km) easy |
| 15 mins easy, 10 mins steady, 20 mins tempo, 15 mins easy | Rest or cross-train | Rest | Long run 16 miles (25.7km), picking up pace over last 10–15 mins |
| 15 mins easy, then 25 mins on a hilly route or circuit, pushing to 10K effort on the climbs, recovering on the flats. Or 15 mins easy then 3–5 long hill repeats (2–3 mins each) on a shallow hill at 10K effort, recovering at a jog, no rest. If doing Parkrun on Saturday, do Saturday's run instead | Rest | 40 mins easy, or Parkrun | Mid-long run 10 miles (16km), picking up to MP or a little quicker over final 4 miles (6.4km). Or a 10-mile (16km) race (not in addition to Parkrun) |
| 15 mins easy, 10 mins steady, 25 mins tempo, 10 mins easy | Rest or cross-train | Rest | Long run 18 miles (29km). Duration no longer than 3 hrs 15 mins. Or equivalent in predicted duration on trail |
| 15 mins easy, then 4 x 6–7 mins at LT pace with 90 secs rest between reps. Surge to faster pace for last min of each rep | Rest | 15 mins easy, then 25 mins on a hilly route or circuit, pushing to 10K effort on the climbs, recovering on the flats. Or 15 mins easy then 3–5 long hill repeats (2–3 mins each) on a shallow hill at 10K effort, recovering at a jog, no rest | 90 mins easy |

| Week | Phase | Monday | Tuesday | Wednesday | |
|------|-------|--------|---------|-----------|---|
| 11 | Development | Rest | 15 mins easy, then 3 x 9–10 mins at LT pace with 2 mins rest | Rest | |
| 12 | Development | Rest | 50 mins easy | Rest | |
| 13 | Specific | Rest | 30 mins very easy | Rest | |
| 14 | Specific | Rest | 60 mins easy | Rest | |
| 15 | Specific | Rest | 40 mins steady | Rest | |
| 16 | Specific | Rest | 30 mins very easy | Rest | |
| 17 | Specific | Rest | 10 mins easy, 25–30 mins tempo, 2 mins rest, then 5 x 60 secs at 1-mile–3K pace with 60 secs rest between reps | Rest | |
| 18 | Taper | Rest | 50 mins easy plus 3–5 x 15-sec strides | Rest | |
| 19 | Taper | Rest | 40 mins easy plus 3 x 15-sec strides | Rest | |
| 20 | Taper | Rest | 20–30 mins easy or rest | Rest | |

| Thursday | Friday | Saturday | Sunday |
|---|---|---|---|
| 40 mins steady | 30 mins easy plus 3–5 x 15-sec strides | Rest | Half-marathon race |
| 15 mins easy, then 'Unders and Overs': alternate 60 secs just below LT pace with 30 secs a little faster for 4 sets (6 mins in total per set) x 3 sets, with 2 mins 30 secs rest between sets | Rest or cross-train | Rest | Long run 20 miles (32km). Duration no longer than 3 hrs 30 mins |
| 5–7-mile (8–11.3km) progression run: start easy, pick up to MP and last 2 miles (3.2km) HMP | Rest | 40 mins easy plus 4 x 10-sec hill sprints | 10 miles (16km) easy, or 80–90 mins on trail, or rest |
| 15 mins easy, 30 mins tempo, 10 mins easy | 30 mins very easy | Rest | 3 miles (4.8km) easy then 4 x 15 mins MP with 1 mile (1.6km) easy between each block, then 2 miles (3.2km) easy |
| 10 mins easy then alternating 2 mins MP, 1 min LT pace for 9 mins. Jog for 5 mins and repeat x 2 more sets | Rest | 30–40 mins MP plus 35 x 15-sec strides, or Parkrun | 16 miles (25.7km) easy |
| 15 mins easy then 'Mile Winders': 1st mile at approx. MP, then each subsequent mile 3–10 secs quicker. Aim for 4–5 reps with 90 secs rest between | 30 mins very easy | Rest | Long run 20 miles (32km) easy. Aim to run 2nd half a little faster than first half by starting out easy. Duration no longer than 3 hrs 30 mins. DRESS REHEARSAL |
| 7–8 miles (11.3–12.9km) easy | 30 mins steady | Rest | 2-hr long run with progression: 30 mins easy, 30 mins MP, 15 mins easy, 15 mins MP, 10 mins easy, 10 mins HMP, 10 mins easy |
| 10 mins easy, then 5 mins LT pace, 2 mins easy, 5 mins LT pace, 2 mins easy, 2 mins 5K pace, 5 mins easy | 30 mins easy or rest | Rest | 90 mins easy |
| 5 miles (8km) steady with surge to MP or HMP for 1 minute at the end of each 1 mile (1.6km) | Rest | Rest | 30 mins easy, 30 mins MP |
| 4 miles (6.4km) easy with last 1 mile (1.6km) MP | Rest | 20–30 mins easy or rest | Race day |

# Minimalist | First–timer ▸ Weeks 1–10

| Week | Phase | Monday | Tuesday | Wednesday | |
|------|-------|--------|---------|-----------|---|
| 1 | Foundation | Rest | 40 mins easy plus 4 x 10-sec hill sprints | Rest | |
| 2 | Foundation | Rest | 40 mins easy plus 4 x 10-sec hill sprints | Rest | |
| 3 | Foundation | Rest | 40 mins easy plus 5 x 10-sec hill sprints | Rest | |
| 4 | Foundation | Rest | 40 mins easy plus 5 x 10-sec hill sprints | Rest | |
| 5 | Foundation | Rest | 40 mins easy plus 6 x 10-sec hill sprints | Rest | |
| 6 | Foundation | Rest | 40 mins easy plus 4 x 15-sec flat sprints | Rest | |
| 7 | Foundation | Rest | 40 mins easy plus 6 x 10-sec hill sprints | Rest | |
| 8 | Foundation | Rest | 40 mins easy plus 4 x 15-sec flat sprints | Rest | |
| 9 | Development | Rest | 50 mins easy | Rest | |
| 10 | Development | Rest | 50 mins easy plus 3–5 x 15-sec strides | Rest | |

| Thursday | Friday | Saturday | Sunday |
|---|---|---|---|
| 40 mins easy with surges of 30 secs every 5th minute (8 in total) | Rest or cross-train | Rest | Long run 12 miles (19.3km) easy (or no more than 120 mins) |
| 15 mins easy, then alternate 30 secs easy/30 secs 1-mile–3K pace x 8. 15 mins easy | Rest or cross-train | Rest | Long run 13 miles (20.9km) easy (or no more than 130 mins) |
| 15 mins easy, then 6 x 1 min at 3–5K pace with 1-min rest between. Jog 5 mins, then 10 mins tempo. If doing Parkrun, do Saturday's session instead | Rest or cross-train | Parkrun or 30 mins steady | Mid-long run 8 miles (12.9km) easy or 80 mins trail |
| 60 mins easy | Rest or cross-train | Rest | Long run 14 miles (22.5km) (or no more than 140 mins) |
| 15 mins easy, then 4 x 2 mins at 5K pace with 2 mins rest between reps, then 10 mins tempo | Rest or cross-train | Rest | Long run 15 miles (24km) easy (or no more than 150 mins) |
| 45 mins easy, including 6–8 x 30–45-sec hill reps at 5K effort, with untimed recoveries then 10 mins tempo | Rest or cross-train | 8 miles (12.9km) easy (or no more than 80 mins) | 7 miles (11.3km) steady (or no more than 60 mins) |
| 15 mins easy, then 10 mins tempo. Then 3 mins, 2 mins, 1 min at 3–5K pace with 90-sec rest between reps. Jog 5 mins then 10 mins tempo | Rest or cross-train | Rest | Long run 16 miles (25.7km), picking up pace over last 10–15 mins (or no more than 165 mins) |
| 15 mins easy, 10 mins steady, 20 mins tempo, 15 mins easy. If doing Parkrun, do Saturday's session instead | Rest or cross-train | Parkrun or 40 mins easy | Mid-long run 8 miles (12.9km) easy or 80 mins on trail |
| 15 mins easy, then 20 mins on a hilly route or circuit, pushing to 10K effort on the climbs, recovering on the flats. Or 15 mins easy then 3–5 long hill repeats (90–120 secs each) on a shallow hill at 10K effort, recovering at a jog, no rest. If doing Parkrun on Saturday, do Saturday's run instead | Rest or cross-train | Rest | Long run 17 miles (27.4km) easy. Duration no longer than 3 hrs |
| 15 mins easy, then 4 x 6 mins at LT pace with 90 secs rest between reps. Surge to faster pace for last 30 secs of each rep | Rest or cross-train | 15 mins easy, 10 mins steady, 25 mins tempo, 10 mins easy | 75–90 mins easy |

| Week | Phase | Monday | Tuesday | Wednesday | |
|------|-------|--------|---------|-----------|---|
| 11 | Development | Rest | 20 mins easy, 20 mins goal HMP | Rest | |
| 12 | Development | Rest | 50 mins easy | Rest | |
| 13 | Specific | Rest | 30 mins very easy | Rest | |
| 14 | Specific | Rest | 60 mins easy | Rest | |
| 15 | Specific | Rest | 40 mins steady | Rest | |
| 16 | Specific | Rest | 30 mins very easy | Rest | |
| 17 | Specific | Rest | 10 mins easy, 20–25 mins tempo, 2 mins rest, then 5 x 45 secs at 1-mile–3K pace, with 45 secs rest between reps | Rest | |
| 18 | Taper | Rest | 40 mins easy plus 3–5 x 15-sec strides | Rest | |
| 19 | Taper | Rest | 40 mins easy plus 3 x 15-sec strides | Rest | |
| 20 | Taper | Rest | 20–30 mins easy or rest | Rest | |

| Thursday | Friday | Saturday | Sunday |
|----------|--------|----------|--------|
| 40 mins steady | 30 mins easy plus 3–5 x 15-sec strides | Rest | Half-marathon race |
| 15 mins easy, then 3 x 8–9 mins at LT pace with 2 mins rest | Rest or cross-train | Rest | Long run 18 miles (29km). Duration no longer than 3 hrs 15 mins. DRESS REHEARSAL |
| 5–7-mile (8–11.3km) progression run: start easy, pick up to MP and last 2 miles (3.2km) HMP | Rest or cross-train | 40 mins easy plus 4 x 10-sec hill sprints | 10 miles (16km) easy, or 80–90 mins on trail, or rest |
| 15 mins easy, 25 mins tempo, 10 mins easy | Rest or cross-train | Rest | 15 miles (24km) progression run: start out very easy, pick up pace at 5 miles (8km) and again at 10 miles (16km) |
| 10 mins easy then alternating 2 mins MP, 1 min LT pace for 6 mins. Jog for 5 mins and repeat x 2 more sets | 30 mins very easy | Rest | Long run 19–20 miles (30.6–32km) easy. Duration no longer than 3 hrs 30 mins |
| 15 mins easy then 'Mile Winders': 1st mile at approx. MP, then each subsequent mile 3–10 secs quicker. Aim for 4 reps with 90 secs rest between reps | Rest or cross-train | 30 mins easy plus 3 x 20-sec flat sprints | 10 miles (16km) easy or 80–90 mins on trail |
| 5–6 miles (8–9.7km) easy | 30 mins steady | Rest | 3 miles (4.8km) easy then 3–4 x 15 mins MP with 1 mile (1.6km) easy between each block, then 2 miles (3.2km) easy |
| 10 mins easy, then 5 mins LT pace, 2 mins easy, 5 mins LT pace, 2 mins easy, 2 mins 5K pace, 5 mins easy | 30 mins easy or rest | Rest | 80–90 mins easy |
| 5 miles (8km) steady with surge to MP or HMP for 1 min at the end of each 1 mile (1.6km) | Rest | Rest | 30 mins easy, 20 mins MP |
| 4 miles (6.4km) easy with last 1 mile (1.6km) MP | Rest | 20–30 mins easy or rest | Race day |

# THE
# PRACTICALITIES

# 5

# GETTING OUT THERE

## The how, when, where (and who with) of making training happen

Running is already part of your lifestyle, so I imagine you are invested in fitting it in. This makes things so much easier, because it skips (or at least minimises) the internal 'shall I go running?' debate, taking you straight to '*when* shall I go running?' or '*where* shall I go running?' That said, you may find that marathon training requires you to alter your usual running regime – for example, track training with the club is replaced by solo tempo runs, or Parkrun only fits in once a month, not weekly. This means some discipline and planning is required to ensure you don't 'default' to the familiar and miss important marathon-training sessions.

### The value of routine

A study published in the *British Journal of Social Psychology* tracked a group of runners training for a marathon over a one-year period. They found that working out how, when and where they were going to do their training made it more likely to happen. Establishing routine is not so much about always having to go at the same time of day (although there's nothing wrong with that) as about being organised and aware of what needs to be done to get out of the door.

Think about circumstances in the past that have caused you to miss sessions. Are skipped runs mostly due to tiredness? Conflicting demands on your time? No one to go with? Identifying what gets in the way of sticking to your plan is the key to making adjustments that will overcome these obstacles.

Work out how you'll fit meals or snacks in around your runs. Make sure your kit is clean and easily accessible (have it laid out ready to put on, or packed in your bag, ideally). Charge your watch or phone. Have your preferred playlist or podcast downloaded. Make your arrangements with other runners, if you're buddying up. I always check the next couple of weeks of my training plan, so that I can swap things around if something's come up that I hadn't originally factored in.

## Finding routes

You will already have some favourite running routes in your area, but with more frequent – and longer – runs on the cards, you could soon find yourself craving some variety.

One of my favourite methods is to get a train or bus somewhere and run home. There's something psychologically cheering about one-way long runs, with every step bringing you closer to home. Don't just stick to roads and pavements (more on running surfaces on p. 93) – there are parks, playing fields, public footpaths, named trails (usually well signposted on the ground, as well as easy to follow on a map), country parks, traffic-free cycleways and towpaths out there. Rivers and canals are great for linear out-and-back runs.

Technology is well placed to help you find new routes. Apps that allow you to devise a route are particularly useful when you are aiming to go a set distance. I like Plotaroute, but there are many other options, including MapMyRun and Strava (*see* Resources). Some apps allow you to plot a route that avoids busy roads and sticks to green space where possible.

Other runners are another limitless source of route inspiration – be that in real life or via technology that enables you to view and upload their routes. I'm always surprised by the number of local runners who've come along on a group run and exclaimed 'I never knew this path was here!'

Running with others also alleviates anxiety about getting lost, or at least makes it more fun if it happens...

## RUN COMMUTING

Using your journey to and/or from work to clock up some miles is great use of time as well as being kinder to the environment, not to mention your wallet. It can take time to find the best route – apps and maps can help, but you won't really know what works best until you've tried a few options. Where possible, avoid running alongside heavy traffic to reduce your exposure to air pollution. And make sure you invest in a comfortable rucksack (see p. 125).

When I run commuted, I took my work clothes and shower gear for the week in on a Monday (without running). Then Tuesday to Thursday, I ran to the office, got showered and changed, and took public transport home. If your workplace doesn't have shower facilities, perhaps there's a gym or health club close by that does. Alternatively, you could take public transport to work, leave your work clothes there and run home. I used my run commute for easy runs only – dodging pedestrians and getting stuck at traffic lights isn't ideal during quality workouts.

## Surface tension

The routes you choose determine – at least to some extent – what's underfoot. Whether you're a trail enthusiast or run exclusively on roads, you'll know that terrain makes a difference to your running experience. An even surface is less challenging to your stability and agility than is a slippery or uneven one, or one with many obstacles like tree roots and rabbit holes; a straight road is less challenging than a twisting single-track path.

Different surfaces also vary in their level of firmness and 'bounce', which impacts on how much energy is absorbed by the terrain rather than returned to the foot. Compare running on a springy athletic track with an energy-sapping sandy beach.

So what type of surface is best? Of course, you have to factor in the surface you'll be running on in your race, because you want to feel comfortable on it. But I recommend that for the sake of both body and mind, you run on a range of different surfaces.

It's often claimed that running on softer surfaces reduces impact. In fact, the impact forces are virtually the same regardless of whether you are running on grass or a concrete pavement. This is because the brain adjusts the muscles' 'stiffness' in anticipation to the density of the surface (basing its response on previous experiences, from the last stride to previous runs). The firmer the surface, the less stiff it will make the muscles – and vice versa. This is known as 'muscle tuning'. Shoes play a role in this, too – so while spongy, soft shoes might *seem* like they're cushioning impact, the picture is more complex, with interactions between the body, the shoe and the surface influencing the outcome.

## One for the road

So, why not just stick to easily accessible, reliable roads? The issue is not with their firmness, but their uniformity. On a road, the exact same stresses are placed on the same muscles, bones and joints with every step. When you run on a more varying surface, like a dirt trail or grassy field, running becomes less metronomic. Every step is a little different, which subtly changes the way the load is experienced by the musculoskeletal system. This may be why people tend to suffer less delayed-onset muscle soreness (DOMS) from long trail runs than from road ones. One study found that an uneven surface with variations of 2.5cm (1in) in height resulted in an increase in the variability of step width and length of 27 per cent and 26 per cent, respectively. The effort involved in coping with changing, uneven terrain also helps strengthen the muscles and connective tissue in a more holistic way, as well as challenging your balance and stability, which in turn, can contribute to a lower risk of injury. The study mentioned above found that the uneven surface increased the workload of the ankle musculature by around 20 per cent compared to flat ground.

I'm not suggesting avoiding asphalt or concrete – it's the surface most runners train on and indeed, most marathons take place on roads. But just as you wouldn't train for the marathon by only doing long runs, don't restrict yourself to only one surface.

## Hitting the trails

Getting out on to the trails is an important part of marathon training for me, because it offers a shift of focus. I find that running off-road requires me to engage more with my surroundings – climbing over stiles, opening and closing gates, edging around path-wide puddles and occasionally stopping to admire the view – which is mentally refreshing. A whole host of studies on green exercise (exercise in natural surroundings) show that it can be psychologically more uplifting than exercise in urban areas or indoors. On the roads, it's easy to get fixated with pace and spend the whole time glancing at your watch. But on the soft, uneven or undulating terrain of the trails, you'll soon find yourself having to abandon any hopes of a constant pace.

One study found that the energy cost of running at a specific pace on an irregular surface was 10 per cent greater than on a level one. So instead of trying to maintain the same pace you would expect to achieve on tarmac, focus on effort level instead. If it's meant to be an easy run, then make sure it *feels* easy. I tend to use off-road terrain mostly for easy runs and for some of my long runs, rather than for sessions in which a specific pace is required, like speedwork. If you are taking on a trail marathon, however, you should consider doing some of your tempo runs, long intervals and race-pace work off-road, too.

## On track

At the other extreme of the surface spectrum from trail lies the athletics track. Designed specifically for running fast, it is level, even and offers huge energy return. The track is ideal for speedwork, drills and short time trials, with its controlled environment (no dogs trotting out in front of you or roads to cross) and easily measurable distances. It can be especially useful in winter, when dark evenings might put you off running in parks and on quiet streets. And there's the added seasonal benefit that as you get warm, you can strip a layer off and leave it close by. But access to a track is by no means essential for any runner, including a marathoner in training. Level paths or circuits on short grass or tarmac work just as well.

# Five tips for novice trail runners

1. If you don't run off-road at the moment but plan to include it in your marathon training, begin with easier surface options, such as a well-worn towpath, woodland trail or playing field. More challenging (often termed 'technical') terrain requires greater agility, experience and confidence.
2. One of the best pieces of trail-running advice I ever read came from the late Caballo Blanco, the Copper Canyon-dwelling ultrarunner who featured in *Born to Run* (Christopher McDougall). 'If you're wondering whether to take one step or two, take three,' he said.
3. Don't look down at your feet. Look at the trail a few metres or yards ahead of you to anticipate how you might need to adjust your stride.
4. Get used to breaking your rhythm. Accept that your pace will speed up and slow down in response to the terrain.
5. Try to relax. This is easier said than done on ever-changing terrain, but being tense wastes energy and tires you out more quickly.

## Run of the mill

There are parallels between the athletics track and the treadmill in terms of the reliable surface, measurability and safe, consistent environment. I'll be honest – I'm not a big fan of running on the treadmill, but I was certainly grateful to have access to one when I was training for a marathon through a bitterly cold – and more to the point, icy – winter. There are other advantages; if you do a tempo run, setting the treadmill at your goal pace, there's no slacking off as you tire, unlike when you're running outside. The incline function is also useful, for hill repeats or for simulating an undulating run.

Avoid doing too much of your training on the treadmill, however. A 2020 study concluded that while it was 'comparable' to running on outdoor surfaces, treadmill running subtly changed some aspects of runners' biomechanics: ground contact time tended to be longer (harnessing less elastic energy) and peak propulsive force (the force applied to the ground during 'take off') lower.

There are also slight differences in the physiological response to treadmill running. A 2019 study found that at easy running paces, heart rate and RPE were lower on the treadmill compared to running at the same pace outdoors, but at faster paces, these variables were higher during treadmill running. This could be due to the biomechanical differences outlined above, or higher body temperature (since faster running creates more heat, which may be dispersed less efficiently indoors).

## Six ways to use the treadmill

1. Recovery runs. Avoid the common mistake of going too fast on your recovery runs by setting the appropriate pace on the treadmill and sticking to it.
2. A time trial. Your ability to precisely control the environment makes the treadmill a good location for a regular time trial (say, every four to six weeks). Warm up first, then select your time (12 minutes is a good test of endurance) or distance and go for it. Keep a record of your results to monitor progress.
3. Form check. This is especially the case if you have a mirror at the side of or in front of the treadmill. But auditory feedback is also useful for revealing a heavy footed or uneven stride and gives you the chance to experiment with ways of running more lightly and evenly.
4. A tempo run. The treadmill comes into its own for this sustained-pace session – providing a trusty surface and ensuring you maintain your goal pace.
5. Heat acclimatisation. If your marathon will be taking place in hot, humid conditions, you can replicate this by wearing extra clothing or using a heater to raise the temperature of the room. However, do not combine this with tougher training sessions – only easy runs. Read more about adapting to running in the heat on p. 103.
6. Hill work. Undulating runs and longer hill reps work well on the treadmill. (If it's a 'rest' rather than a jog recovery, straddle the treadmill belt rather than putting the incline back down to stop or walk.) The treadmill isn't advisable for hill sprints, though; it takes too long to get the incline and speed to the required level (and the machine may not be able to go fast enough anyway).

# The ups and downs of gradient

Talking of hills, it's worth briefly considering the difference an incline or decline bestows on a session.

Running uphill obviously increases energy demand – the greater the incline, the higher the oxygen cost – due to greater muscle activity, especially from those glutes. But this extra effort has pay-offs. New Zealand sport scientists found that adding uphill training improved time trial performance over 5km (3.1 miles) by 2 per cent. High-intensity efforts had the greatest effect on running economy, while moderate-intensity efforts had the most positive effect on aerobic fitness, neatly demonstrating why it's important to include a range of different types of hill training.

As with uneven or soft surfaces, use effort level rather than pace to judge your effort when you take to the hills.

Unsurprisingly, the energy cost of downhill running is lower than flat or uphill running and again, is related to the extent of the gradient – but only to a certain point. Once a slope becomes very steep, the energy cost rises again, because muscles have to work hard to control your descent. Increased downhill gradients are also associated with a higher loading rate (especially at the knee joint) and impact force, which could raise injury risk.

When you are running downhill, the number one rule is to relax. Try to avoid the temptation to 'brake' by leaning back and sticking your feet too far out in front of you (overstriding). This puts lots of stress on your quads and knees as well as slowing you down. Instead, keep your posture upright (shoulders over hips, hips over feet) and make your strides shorter and quicker. You'll soon hear the difference between the heavy thuds of overstriding and the quieter landings of this nimbler stride.

## When to run

You may not have the luxury of choosing when to run. It may be dictated by where it fits best into your busy life. Nonetheless, research suggests that time of day can affect how your body responds to exercise.

Our bodies have an inbuilt 24-hour clock – known as the circadian rhythm – during which biological parameters including hormone levels, body temperature and power output rise and fall in a predictable way. For example, the 'stress' hormone cortisol is highest in the morning, while body temperature peaks at between 4 and 6 p.m. These fluctuations may affect your body's response to exercise. In one study, overweight people lost more weight when they exercised in the morning, which ties in with the results of a 2019 study on mice that indicated muscle cells are better able to metabolise sugar and fat in the mornings. Other research suggests that runners who struggle with sleep problems should exercise in the morning, because running later in the day may blunt their melatonin response, a hormone associated with readiness to sleep.

Time of day has been shown to impact on athletic performance, too. One study found that the peak power cyclists achieved in a high-intensity workout was 7.6 per cent greater at 6 p.m. than at 2 a.m., 6 a.m., 10 a.m., 2 p.m. or 10 p.m. Indeed, the evidence overall strongly suggests that athletic performance is best in the evening.

Or is it? Well, Tunisian research shows that adaptations to training are greatest when we train at the time of day which we've become most accustomed to. In other words, you get better at what you practise the most. This also raises the important issue of consistency. People who exercise at a regular time of day are more consistent (amassing more training time overall) than those who exercise at more random times.

## Larks and owls

As well as circadian rhythms, we each have our own chronotype (our natural inclination towards being energetic or lethargic at different times of the day). Perhaps you see yourself as a 'morning person' or a 'night owl'. This, too, plays a role in what time of day is most conducive to your running because you respond best (as measured by rate of perceived exertion and fatigue rating) to exercise when the timing of the workout chimes with your chronotype.

One study measured cortisol levels (a biomarker for stress) during high-intensity morning exercise in larks and owls. Cortisol levels peak in the morning, regardless of exercise. But the study found that while cortisol rose after exercise in both morning and evening types, the former experienced far *less* elevation (both immediately post-exercise and up to an hour later) suggesting they coped better with the morning workout due to their chronotype.

Conversely, rate of perceived exertion *rises* when you have to exercise at a non-accustomed time. One study found that 'morning' cyclists rated an identical workout as more challenging when they had to do it in the evening, compared to their usual time of day.

What does this all mean to you? Well, your best performances are likely to be at the time of day you're most accustomed to running at. However, the chances are that your marathon will take place in the morning. So, if you are an owl, you should schedule some long runs – and races – on mornings between now and race day to 'acclimatise' to exercising at this time of day. Try to precede these runs with an earlier night than usual so you don't feel too fatigued. Judicious use of caffeine on waking up might help you feel more ready for morning exercise.

Intriguingly, research does suggest that elite endurance exercisers – including distance runners, cyclists and triathletes – are more likely to be 'morning' types. It's not clear whether this is due to larks being drawn to activities that typically take place in the morning, or whether night owls simply don't do as well in endurance sport because of scheduling conflicts.

Ultimately, remember that the biggest influencer on performance is training itself – so fitting your sessions in where you can is far more important than finding the perfect time of day for them.

## Who to run with

One of the best things about running is that it is a totally independent pursuit. You don't need anyone to make it happen except yourself. But as with so many aspects of training, variety – solo runs, buddy runs, group or club runs – offers the widest benefits. A training partner or group can make running more sociable, widen your repertoire of routes and be a valuable source of advice, support and tips. It's also much easier to get through tough workouts, such as intervals and hill work, when you've got someone to run with – or chase. On a practical level, it's also helpful to have another pair of eyes for when you are counting reps or timing an effort. But remember it's *you* who is running this marathon; don't get drawn into 'racing' on easy runs and long runs, running extra sessions (or races) that aren't in your plan or pushing too hard simply to keep up with others.

The ideal running partner(s) would be roughly the same speed as you. It can be risky to buddy up with someone faster; however well intentioned their offer to run with you, you are almost certainly going to end up going too fast, jeopardising either the run itself or your recovery from it. Keep an eye on your pace, heart rate or RPE to ensure that it is appropriate for the type of run you're doing. It should not differ from what you'd expect if you were running alone.

## Going clubbing

Gone are the days when the majority of runners belonged to a club. A 2021 government survey found that more than 7 million people in the UK claim to run at least twice a month – yet there are just 172,000 official club members. (Many more are members of non-affiliated and informal groups.) If you're not one of them, should you be?

Clubs vary widely in terms of their ethos, membership base and activities. I've been a member of half a dozen clubs over the years, and they were all completely different. I've been among the fastest runners at one club and the slowest at another! The only way to find out if a club is the right fit for you is to go along and try it out. Most offer a couple of 'no obligation' sessions before you need to join. The potential benefits include great coaching, group runs and people to run with or against, as well as opportunities to compete for the club (and discounted race entry). There can be drawbacks, though: rigid and repetitive training, less flexibility about when and where you run, excessive volume or intensity and pressure to race too often. If you're already into marathon training and things are going well, I'd advise delaying joining a club until after the race, when you're less tied to a specific training regime. But if you're struggling for motivation, support, routes and running buddies, why not give it a go? You might find your perfect running partner!

## Going solo

While it's nice to have company on some of your runs, I recommend doing at least some of them – particularly long runs – alone. It will help you tune into your pace better and, owing to the lack of distraction, will probably feel harder, which is good for building confidence and mental strength. But do consider your personal safety, especially if you're running in remote, unpeopled or unfamiliar areas or running in the dark. Here are some top tips:

- Run in areas where there are other people, and at times of the day when there are more people around; avoid poorly lit areas in the evening and early morning.
- Let someone know where you're going, and roughly when you'll be back. If there's no one home, leave a note or send a text or message.
- Consider taking your phone, even if you switch it to airplane mode to avoid interruptions. On long runs, you might want to take a bankcard or some money, in case you need to bail out for some reason and need funds for transport home or sustenance.
- If you wear earphones when you're out running, keep the volume low enough to be aware of your surroundings and the people or traffic around you.
- Avoid routes in the dark that you haven't run in daylight first. Not only are you far less likely to end up on an unlit narrow lane or isolated industrial estate, but you'll also be more aware of any hazards along the way, such as cracked paving, bollards or slippery drain covers.
- On trail routes far from roads, carry extra clothing and snacks in case you get lost or the weather changes.

## Running and weather

The weather can make or break a running session. But in marathon training, you need to learn to cope with all eventualities, not just to get the training done in the timescale you have but also because you never know what weather you'll face come race day. The old adage about there being no such thing as inappropriate weather, only inappropriate clothing, holds true – but there are some other useful strategies to help you cope with the extremes.

## Hot stuff

If the weather turns hot during marathon training, there is an important question to consider. Should you be doing your best to avoid the heat, by training in the early mornings or evenings and choosing shaded routes – or should you be trying to adapt to cope better in the heat? It all depends on the likely conditions come race day.

If it's a given that you'll be racing in hot conditions, acclimatisation is definitely the best option. But allow your body time to adapt, starting with easier, shorter runs in the heat before building up to longer or harder sessions. And there is no need to seek out heat on every run. Experts reckon that adaptation occurs after 10–14 days. *See* p. 97 for advice on treadmill 'heat runs'.

Lots of studies show that 'pre-cooling' (actively making yourself cooler before you run) is helpful. Tried-and-tested methods include drinking a slushy (a crushed ice drink), having a cold shower or dip, draping an icy towel around your neck and shoulders – or, as seen at the sultry Tokyo Olympics, putting an icepack under your cap. Keep out of the sun for as long as you can before you start running and once you're on the move, drink plenty of fluids but also pour some cold water over your head at regular intervals to dissipate heat.

A strange but worthwhile heat acclimatisation strategy to consider is taking a hot bath after your runs. Researchers at the University of Bangor found that six days of post-run hot baths successfully lowered body temperature at rest and during exertion, leading to an improved 5K time trial performance. The runners bathed for 40 minutes, but the researchers say 20 minutes will still be beneficial. Some preliminary evidence also suggests that this practice may enhance training adaptations and boost the immune system.

## Cold comfort

If you're more likely to be facing the big freeze than wall-to-wall sunshine, I'll start with some heartening information. In 2012, French researchers looked at the race-day temperature in relation to the finishing times of 1.8 million marathoners over a 10-year period. They found that a race-day temp of 6.2°C (43.2°F) produced the quickest times. That's pretty chilly. (When they looked at elite finishers, the fastest times were achieved at even lower temperatures.) So cold weather doesn't present as much of a performance challenge as hot weather. Though it can be harder to face.

There's some advice on dressing for cold weather in Chapter 7. But a few training tweaks can help soften the blow, too. I often begin warming up indoors, performing some mobility exercises, jogging on the spot or going up and down stairs so I am already producing some body heat by the time I go outside. Or you might just put your running kit on the radiator before you set off. If you're doing speedwork, consider whether you can swap rest periods for walking or easy jogging, to avoid standing still and getting cold. If it's a long run on a windy day, set off into the headwind so it is behind you on the way home when you're more tired and have been exposed to the elements for longer. In really adverse conditions, consider running loops closer to home rather than tackling a long 'out and back' run, in case you need to bail out. Bear in mind that surfaces are most likely to be icy in the early morning and evening, in which case, if possible, choose trail or grass as it will have more grip than roads and pavements. Finally, don't neglect hydration (even though you may not feel as thirsty) and fuelling on wintry runs. Once you get home, get out of cold or wet kit as soon as you can.

# BE SAFE, BE SEEN

Whether you are running alone or with others, be traffic aware. The golden rule is to make sure you can be seen, but never to assume that you have been. There are two different measurements of visibility: 'perception distance', which is the point at which a driver has spotted something, and 'recognition distance', which is the point at which they've recognised the 'something' as a runner. Even in daylight, wearing fluorescent clothing (yellow, pink or orange) will improve perception distance. But if you're running after dark, you need to go one step further, because reflective materials can increase recognition distance to as much as 200m (220 yards). For maximum effectiveness, the reflective bits should be on your 'moving parts' (the arms and legs), rather than on your trunk, as movement makes them easier to spot. A head or body light is also useful, both for lighting your way and raising your visibility. If you're running on the road, you should face the oncoming traffic unless you are approaching a blind bend, and keep well in (single file, if you're in a pair or group).

# 6
# THE MENTAL MARATHON

## Making use of your grey matter to train and race better

There's an old adage that running is 90 per cent mental. With all the effort you're putting into your training, you may feel sceptical about this. And while no amount of positive thinking, motivation or pain tolerance is going to compensate for a lack of physical preparation, it is true that your brain has a huge influence on the experience – and outcome – of your training and racing. For example, a study from the University of Illinois found that athletes who believed that they could tolerate leg muscle pain did better in a running trial than those who doubted their ability to handle the discomfort. Your mind can be your greatest ally – or your worst enemy. That's why a sports psychologist is now as much a part of an elite athlete's support team as the nutritionist or physio.

I'm not suggesting every common-or-garden marathoner should employ a sports psychologist. But flexing a little mental muscle can help runners manage anxiety, screen out negative thoughts, improve attentional focus, regulate pace and push through discomfort, to name a few benefits. So how can you get your mind onside?

# Go for goals

The brain works best with a clear direction: a goal, a reason for wanting it and a path to getting it. If you haven't already set a goal and decided on a timescale and training plan, do so. One of the reasons this is so important is that it gives every session meaning – placing it within the 'bigger picture'. Working towards goals doesn't always feel good in the moment – for example, running mile repeats isn't pleasurable at the time – but the fact that it is contributing towards your sub-3 hrs 30 mins marathon goal gives it purpose and value, raising your motivation to do it. Without a clear direction, any and every session is expendable and you may soon find yourself losing focus and interest.

A marathon takes time to train for – and the remoteness of that goal on the calendar from the present can make it feel non-urgent and far away. Again, having a plan that takes you from now to race day helps, by filling in all those weeks (that your mind perhaps perceives as 'free') with important training. It can also be motivating to set some interim goals – stepping stones on the journey – that give you something more immediate to work towards and a chance to 'check in' with how you are progressing. But do be wary of letting instant gratification get in the way of long-term gains. Strava kudos and Parkrun PBs are all very nice, but keep your eyes on the prize.

## The ebb and flow of motivation

I love running. But that doesn't mean I set out on every run bursting with enthusiasm, or return feeling on top of the world. Sometimes, running just doesn't work its magic. It feels dull, or hard, or like just another thing to fit into a busy day. You too? Don't worry, it's totally normal (if a little inconvenient during marathon training!) – and it's not worth beating yourself up over.

At times like this, I find it helpful to reflect on my motivation. I ask myself what got me signing up for this particular marathon. Try asking yourself the same question. Did you feel it was finally time to test yourself against the ultimate race distance? Did you move up into a new age group? Did you pledge to run it in memory of someone you loved? Did you want to take what you'd learned from your last effort and smash your

PB? Reminding yourself what got you started on this journey can really help when running loses its lustre.

The other critical thing is to have some support. This is particularly true if it's your first marathon – you need someone you can talk to about the ups and downs of your training. Whether it's a running club buddy, your partner or even your physio, we all need someone with whom to share our successes, hopes, doubts and fears. Social media and online running communities, like Lonely Goat, have proliferated for just this reason and might provide the outlet you need if you can't find it in person.

Here are some useful tricks to have up your sleeve to get you into your trainers when motivation is low.

## Getting yourself out of the door...

- Get up and put your running kit on. Even if you're feeling ambivalent about running, the 'cue' you have presented your brain with will likely nudge you into getting out there. There have been times where I've spent the entire day in my running kit, finally getting out at dusk and wondering why on earth I put it off for so long...
- Runs with an external purpose work a treat for me when I'm struggling with motivation. For example, I've run to the chemist to pick up a prescription, to the library with a rucksack of books to return and to my favourite cafe to meet a friend and walk home. I could have driven or cycled any of these journeys, but running them and ticking off a task or errand at the same time kills two birds with one stone and feels gratifyingly productive.
- Sign up to an interim race. This could either be a way of doing a long run on a planned and marked route with some company, or a proper race. Decide in advance whether you are racing or training. This will be determined largely by where you are in your training plan.
- Promise yourself a reward. I knew a runner who put a pound coin into a tin every time she completed a run. Within a few weeks, she had enough money to treat herself to a new running top. Other running friends always finish long runs with coffee and a big slab of cake. My favourite post-long-run reward is an afternoon nap!
- Play music. Research by Dr Costas Karageorghis, a leading authority on music and running, shows that listening to music can nudge

you into the right frame of mind for a run. Music elevates positive aspects of mood such as excitement and happiness and reduces negative aspects, like tension and fatigue. What kind of music? Anything at all, as long as you like it. A study in 2020 found that when rowers listened to their preferred music during a warm-up, their subsequent performance in a time trial was better than when they listened to no music, or to music they didn't like. Read about the effects of listening to music *during* running on p. 112.

- Arrange to meet someone. A training partner – or group – can be a godsend. It's someone to make plans with, increasing your 'accountability' for showing up. It's someone who can lead you on new and different routes from your usual ones. It's someone to chat to, be it about running or anything else. It's someone to help you through the tough moments and celebrate the joys with. And of course, you are providing all these things for them, too. Read more about running with others on p. 100.

## - Too much?

WHILE IT'S PERFECTLY natural for motivation to ebb and flow, if you find that negative feelings around running persist, it's worth taking stock. Are you overtraining? (*See* 'Signs of burnout and overtraining' on p. 117.) Are you putting too much pressure on yourself? Keep things in perspective – running is meant to be pleasurable and rewarding. I'm not saying training for a marathon isn't demanding – but it should be enhancing your life, not blighting it.

## Can your brain help you run faster?

So, we've talked about harnessing the brain to make training happen – what about its influence on performance? There is strong scientific support for the idea that when it comes to getting every last drop of effort out of yourself, it's the brain that is in the driving seat, not the muscles.

It was Professor Tim Noakes who first proposed a theory that put 'central' (brain) fatigue over 'peripheral' (body) fatigue. His Central Governor Theory (CGT) contends that our capacity to 'endure' in endurance performance is regulated by the brain. When the stress of exercise approaches the limit of what is deemed safe by specific areas within the brain (collectively, the 'central governor'), the brain's motor cortex prevents further muscle recruitment, creating fatigue and discomfort that force you to slow down or stop. I always picture my central governor as an over-zealous little man in a yellow hard hat, lurking in the corner of my brain with a clipboard.

A good illustration of CGT in action is approaching the finish line in a race. Even when your pace has slowed over the last few miles and you feel you have nothing left to give, on seeing that finish line, you can suddenly produce a 400m (440-yard) sprint! If your muscles really were spent, how would that be possible? From a CGT point of view, registering that your run is about to come to an end (in essence, that the 'threat' of excessive exertion is now over), the 'governor' loosens its grip and allows you to recruit more muscles and finish strong.

There's an alternative theory to Noakes's. It has the same central tenet that it's the brain, not the muscles, that regulates or 'governs' endurance performance – but while CGT holds that the process is subconscious, in Professor Samuele Marcora's Psychobiological Model of Endurance Performance, it's conscious. Marcora questions why we would need 'feedback', in the form of fatigue or pain, if we have a central governor that can simply switch off muscle recruitment when it senses we're entering the danger zone.

## The role of perceived effort

Marcora's model postulates that we will engage in a task, like running, until the effort (defined as 'the struggle to continue against a mounting desire to stop') required to do so exceeds the level we are willing – or able – to endure.

Our decisions on pacing and quitting are based primarily on how hard we believe ourselves to be working at any given moment. This isn't about how much pain or discomfort we're feeling, claims Marcora – it's very specifically to do with the level of *effort* we perceive we are putting in. Perceived effort and actual effort are not necessarily the same thing. Take the example of running at a set pace for a prolonged period. At first, the pace feels very comfortable. Then it gets a bit harder, and a bit harder, until at some point, a few hours later, it feels almost impossible to carry on. Your actual effort – in terms of pumping out 10-minute miles – hasn't changed. But your perception of effort has rocketed.

You might interject at this point – *of course fatigue is physiological!* As you get tired, your body sends signals to your brain telling it to slow down or stop. But while Marcora agrees that tired, hurting muscles negatively affect performance, he believes it's because these unpleasant sensations influence perception of effort, rather than through any direct feedback mechanism.

There are a whole host of physiological and psychological factors that can affect perception of effort and thereby performance. Imagine you are coming up to the 17-mile (27.4km) marker in the marathon. When you get there, you realise it's actually the 16-mile (25.7km) marker. This strikes quite a blow and quite possibly, makes you suddenly feel more tired and demotivated. Now imagine that it turns out to be the 18-mile (29km) marker! In this scenario you probably feel energised, and your perception of effort lowers.

A study that Marcora and colleagues did in 2014 demonstrates the power of perception. Cyclists rode to exhaustion while looking at a screen that periodically flashed up human faces, either happy or sad. The images vanished so quickly that they were only registered by the riders on a subconscious level. But those shown the happy faces lasted 12 per cent longer. Why? Improved mood reduces perception of effort.

There is clearly a big difference between believing that the way the brain limits performance is a conscious or subconscious process. But in some respects, whether it's an issue of protection or perception is immaterial. The fact remains that a feeling overcomes us that says 'no more!' – and we want to know how we can stop this happening – or at least delay the point at which it occurs.

## Getting comfortable with being uncomfortable

One thing that has come out of research into the limits of endurance performance and the role of the brain is the finding that elite athletes seem better able to 'suffer' than less experienced athletes. You could argue that the likes of Kipchoge have a natural ability to withstand the pain of extreme effort, but experts believe it's not that they 'feel' less pain, they are just more willing to put up with it in pursuit of their goal than the rest of us.

There are two aspects to pain. Pain threshold is the point at which something is initially perceived as pain. Pain tolerance is the maximum level of perceived pain someone will tolerate. In research at the University of Kent, athletes' tolerance to pain in a general pain test did not correlate with endurance performance – but tolerance to exercise-induced pain did. Subjects who endured greater amounts of pain during a fixed-effort exercise task were generally able to produce faster 10-mile (16km) time trial performances.

It follows, then, that your capacity to 'suffer' or tolerate discomfort or even pain is a key determinant in how close you can get to your physical potential. So, how can you raise the bar on suffering?

Get used to it! Your 'history' of withstanding pain in the past feeds into your ability to tolerate more in the future. Once you've done it before, you're more likely to be able to do it again. And that's where training comes in. From a CGT point of view, exposure to bouts of high-intensity or prolonged effort can 'raise the point' at which your internal health and safety officer flicks the 'off' switch – and reassures the brain that you have been in this particular pain cave before and lived to tell the tale, prompting it to allow you to push that bit harder.

Sessions like fast-finish long runs and progression runs, as well as no-rest interval sessions (where you keep jogging between efforts rather than stopping), are great ways of cranking up the effort level just when you are ready for it to wind down.

## Making running feel easier...

There are ways of lowering – and raising – your perception of effort during running. (And surprisingly, both can be beneficial when it comes to race day.)

The effect of music on performance has been widely studied, and for good reason: more than half of all runners listen to music or other audio while they run. Music can positively affect mood and sensation of effort while running – and even improve performance. In a study at Keele University in 2012, participants reported lower rates of perceived exertion (RPE) and feeling more 'in the zone' when they listened to their chosen music genre, be it classical or death metal.

There's been a lot of research on choosing music of a particular cadence (beats per minute), in order to synchronise or 'entrain' foot strike to music. Some studies have found that this entrainment improves performance, but others have found that the task of entrainment itself is mentally demanding to some. It may be that if you don't naturally 'run to the beat' then attempting to do so is counterproductive. A 2021 study on recreational runners offers support for this contention. First of all, the runners' individual 'typical' cadence was determined. Then they participated in a trial under three conditions. In the first, there was no music. In the second, they were played music and instructed to entrain their footsteps to the beat of the music. In the final scenario, they listened to the same music but were not given any instructions about entrainment. While cadence was higher in both music conditions, stride length and overall speed were only higher when the runners were not told to synchronise their steps.

Part of the reason that music can reduce perception of effort is because it acts as a distraction, drawing you away from the discomfort of pushing yourself. That's why a podcast – no good for synchronising your foot strike or energising your mood – can still be helpful.

Sports psychologists talk about something called 'attentional style' in relation to what we focus on during exercise. In an associative attentional style, you focus on internal stimuli, such as the breath or the rhythm of your feet. In a dissociative style, you pay attention to external stimuli, such as shop windows, your playlist or the conversation of a fellow runner.

It's long been purported that an associative, inward-looking focus is the more successful strategy, and the one more commonly used by accomplished runners. But recent research has contested this – finding that focusing on breathing or the movement of the body actually *worsens* running economy. It may be a little like driving; once you're a seasoned driver, you perform all those different actions – changing gear, looking in the rear-view mirror, steering, braking – without conscious thought. The moment you try to pay conscious attention to what you're doing it feels more complicated and challenging. However, simply tuning in to how your body feels, as in 'body scanning', described on p. 156, rather than on these more automated processes, does not have a negative impact on economy.

What I draw from all this is that we have options as to where we focus our attention – which is a good thing. If you feel you need to distract yourself (from self-doubt, discomfort, or even boredom) during a run, you can look outwards (for example, engage with the crowd or marshals on race day). And when you need to really tune in to your body, you can do that, too. One study found that in training, only 21 per cent of elite runners used solely associative strategies, with 43 per cent using just dissociative and 36 per cent employing both.

If you fancy trying a more subversive approach, you could try swearing your way through your next punishing workout! A study from Keele University found that when subjects had to endure the pain of immersing an arm in iced water, cursing while doing so enabled them to stick it out for longer.

One final thing to consider is caffeine. Countless studies have shown that using caffeine can improve performance. Caffeine acts on the brain, not the muscles, making exercise feel easier, therefore allowing you to push closer to your true limit before you reach the edge of your tolerance for the discomfort you're experiencing. *See* p. 245 for more details.

## ...and harder

I mentioned that strategies that *raise* your perception of effort could also be useful, which I admit, sounds counterintuitive. But for Professor Marcora, things that make running feel a little less comfortable increase the training load, which your brain then adapts to. The key here is restricting such strategies to training and keeping them well away from racing. Think of it like training with a weighted vest that you then throw off on race morning. Runners who feel they 'have' to run with music, for example, could benefit from occasionally leaving the earphones at home and facing the harder prospect of training in silence.

Marcora's research has also shown that preceding physical training with mentally exhausting tasks can ramp up the overall effort required during exercise, since both challenge the brain areas involved in regulating effort and resisting fatigue. For example, in one study, subjects had to perform a laborious 30-minute mental test before taking part in a timed 5K. They fared worse in the time trial after the mental test compared to running 'fresh', even though physiological parameters like oxygen uptake, blood lactate and heart rate didn't appear to be affected.

This suggested to Marcora that mental fatigue could have just as detrimental an effect on endurance performance as physical fatigue, by raising perceived exertion. So, he got the subjects to introduce pre-workout mental training exercises into their regime regularly. The result? He found that their performance in the subsequent exercise test improved, indicating that mental training had a 'training effect', just as adding more physical training would.

Even if you have no intention of adding mentally-fatiguing exercise to your regime, one point to take away from this is that it's important to do your best to avoid mental fatigue in the days leading up to your race, as it can have a genuinely negative effect on performance. And bear in mind that we are not as conscious of mental fatigue as we are of physical tiredness.

## Pain is inevitable, suffering is optional

There's another way to draw out your best performances. Rather than looking to reduce your perception of effort, you *raise* the amount of effort you are willing to invest to succeed in the task, so the suffering becomes less of an issue. In essence, you make yourself want it more.

One of the most powerful effects on our willingness to suffer during exercise is the presence of others. In one study, cyclists who were pitted against an avatar were able to perform faster in a time trial than in the same test performed alone. Another study, from New York University, found that runners performed best in races that featured their known rivals. The researchers suggest that the presence of a rival raises the psychological stakes, and increases the amount of effort a runner is willing to put in. The average improvement equated to running eight seconds faster per mile (five seconds faster per km). That's three-and-a-half minutes over a marathon!

But I think it's important to use this strategy sparingly. For example, if you're meant to be doing an easy long run, then getting competitive with a fellow runner isn't helpful at all. But if you're meant to be knocking out some high-intensity intervals, it could be. The same goes for race day – while you might usefully try to latch on to someone in the last few miles as a way of motivating yourself to keep pushing, avoid letting your competitive streak overcome you from the outset and throwing your well-prepared race plan into the wind.

An audience has also been shown to help athletes raise their game. Research in the journal *Social Cognitive and Affective Neuroscience* in 2018 found that when people know they are being observed, parts of the brain associated with social awareness and reward are stimulated. This may go some way to explaining why you can pull performances out of the bag in races that you cannot achieve in training.

It's a given that on race day there will be an audience of sorts, but you may want to consider the type of race you choose if you feel that having a large, loving crowd might bring out strengths that you wouldn't muster in a smaller, less well supported race. (I once did a marathon in Orkney and beautiful as it was, away from the start and finish areas the audience mostly consisted of a couple of farmers leaning on a gate.)

Another tactic for increasing your willingness to suffer in the moment is to remember past experiences when you didn't. Psychologist Robert Wicks coined the term 'sweet disgust' to describe the feeling of disappointment or irritation at yourself for quitting that drives you to do better next time. Harness it to increase your motivation and reframe your perception of effort.

In his book *What I Talk About When I Talk About Running*, Haruki Murakami uses the phrase 'pain is inevitable, suffering is optional' – and this captures the concept perfectly. The pain is an inevitable part of pushing yourself to the maximum, but whether you choose to see this as suffering – or something else – is up to you.

All in all then, there are as many ways to train your mind to support your marathon as there are ways to train your body. You can read more about race-day tricks in Section 5.

# SIGNS OF BURNOUT AND OVERTRAINING

Runners often think that overtraining is just the territory of elites. How can a mere recreational runner succumb to such a thing? But overtraining simply means that, over an extended period of time, you have been attempting to do more than your body can cope with, sending it into a sort of overdrive. It can happen to anyone. If the list of symptoms below strikes a chord with you, take five to seven days off running. Eat healthily and get lots of rest and sleep. If you have physical symptoms, you may want to visit your GP for the peace of mind of ruling out any underlying medical problem or illness, such as anaemia.

I understand that you will be worried about losing fitness, but ignoring these symptoms and continuing to train as you are (or worse still, seeing it as a sign that you aren't working hard enough and pushing even harder) is likely to result in your performance deteriorating far more, and for far longer. It may be that a few days off is all you need to recharge, or you may find that you need to downsize your schedule or balance it with better nutrition and sleep patterns.

Signs of overtraining are:
- Poor performance or unusually high heart rate or RPE during training;
- Depressed mood or irritability;
- Lack of motivation;
- Consistently raised resting heart rate, 5–10bpm above normal;
- Recurring colds, sore throats, mouth ulcers or other signs of suppressed immune system;
- Sleep problems (not being able to sleep, interrupted sleep, difficulty getting up);
- Increased muscle soreness;
- General fatigue;
- Fluctuating appetite and weight (weight loss and appetite loss are common, but some runners may subconsciously be trying to increase sapped energy levels by eating more);
- Irregular or absent periods in menstruating women.

# 7

# RUNNING SHOES AND KIT

## What to wear for training and racing

Footwear has always been a hot topic in running, and no more so than in the last few years – since 2016, to be precise. This is when shoe giant Nike introduced its first carbon-fibre plate shoe, the Vaporfly 4%. Since then, every distance-running world record – male and female, from 5K to marathon – has been broken. In 2019, athletes wearing shoes from the Vaporfly range won 86 per cent of all podium spots at 12 major marathons. Nike's claims of a 4 per cent improvement in running economy and a corresponding 2 per cent improvement in performance time have stood up under scientific scrutiny. Other brands rushed to produce their own 'super shoes' to get a piece of the action. They are now commonplace.

You might assume that getting a pair of these lace-up ergogenic aids should be a top priority for an aspiring marathoner. That's certainly the way many athletes – elite and recreational – feel; that they 'have' to have them in order to compete on a level playing field. It's the same *'but everyone's doing it!'* argument used by cyclists caught taking illicit drugs in the Tour de France (though at time of going to press, carbon plate shoes are still legal!). But the truth is, there is and always will be a range of footwear on people's feet, catering for different preferences and budgets. The hefty price tag of carbon plate running shoes certainly rules them out for many runners.

I have to confess they aren't on my shopping list. It's partly because I feel they're a bit of a cop-out. If I go for a PB and I'm wearing shoes that have been proven to improve performance, then if I achieve my goal, I'll be wondering if it was me or the shoes.

There are other reasons why I haven't succumbed to the lure of go-faster shoes. First, after decades of experimentation – from motion control to minimalist, I now have a very clear picture of what I want from my running shoes – and these shoes don't tick my boxes. Personal preference, as unscientific as it might sound, is an important factor in choosing the right footwear, as you'll read in a moment.

Second, these shoes are designed for running on flat, even surfaces. Although that might fit the bill for many road marathons, it doesn't make up the bulk of my training terrain so they'd spend a lot of time in the cupboard.

And finally, we don't yet know if there are long-term ill effects from wearing carbon-plate running shoes. One thing the stiff, curved sole of the shoe does is reduce the foot's natural side-to-side motion (in order to optimise forward motion). Does that mean lateral stability weakens over time? Does limiting the foot's natural spring reduce its capacity to absorb shock? Anecdotally, I've noticed a lot of Achilles tendon and plantar fascia issues in runners wearing carbon plate shoes. But at the moment we simply don't know if there's any injury risk associated with their use.

The excitement over a shoe that seems to enhance performance has taken the spotlight off the more commonly debated shoe topic – injury prevention.

## Running shoes and injury

Among the claims that running shoe companies make about their wares are that they can help 'correct' shortcomings in your biomechanics (such as overpronation), cushion you from the impact of hard surfaces, help you run more 'efficiently', strengthen your feet and protect you from injuries. Can they? Well, in 2015, a landmark study in the *British Journal of Sports Medicine* reviewed a wealth of research on running footwear and injuries and concluded that there was no evidence to support the oft-claimed link between pronation and increased injury risk; nor could they substantiate claims that cushioning prevented injuries.

A year earlier, a US trial with over 7000 subjects found no evidence to support the prescription of specific shoe types – stability, cushioned or motion control (known as 'shoe shop theory') – according to foot morphology (e.g. flat feet or high arches). There was no difference in injury rates among people with different foot types, nor did being prescribed the 'right' type of shoe for their foot type offer any protection from injury compared to a randomly prescribed shoe. More recently, a study published in the *Journal of Athletic Training* (December 2020) concluded: 'it is possible that the role of running shoe technology in injury prevention has been largely overrated.'

This isn't to say that running shoes are useless or that we should all go barefoot. But it does raise two points. One, that many of the claims made about how shoes can protect or correct your feet are exaggerated, or plain wrong. Two, that having shoes 'prescribed' for you, based on foot type or indeed, a broader assessment, has not been shown to be protective against injury. It turns out that it's perfectly possible to have a high arch and still overpronate like a flat-footer. The days of the 'wet footprint test' or jumping on a treadmill to be filmed from the knee down and told by the shop assistant what shoe you should be wearing are gone. See pp. 184–5 for more on the relationship between injury and footwear.

## Choosing the right shoe

So, what criteria *should* you use to choose your running footwear? Comfort, says Dr Benno Nigg, author of the 2015 study. Much as this might sound like the sort of advice your nan would give you ('Is it comfortable, dear?') Nigg is one of the world's most eminent biomechanists and author of an entire book called *The Biomechanics of Sports Shoes*.

Critics have contested that 'comfort' is a woolly term. It could be taken to mean that your running shoes should feel as squishy and familiar as your favourite slippers. But Nigg talks about comfort in relation to what he calls the 'preferred movement path'. This refers to the fact that your body 'wants' to move in a specific and unique pattern, which is shaped by your particular anatomy – some shoes will facilitate this better than others. It doesn't mean everyone should wear minimalist shoes – it could be that your preferred movement path is least hampered by a chunkier option. But it does bring home the point that the person who knows best about what shoes are right for you is you.

I still recommend going to a specialist running shop to buy your shoes. Putting a wide range of shoes through what Nigg calls your 'comfort filter' is the best way to find out what suits you. Plus you can get good advice on fit from a reputable store. Or if you liked one particular model of shoe that is no longer available, they might be able to suggest a similar alternative.

## WHEN SHOULD I REPLACE MY SHOES?

You'll often hear that running shoes should be replaced every 300–500 miles (480–800km). There is no scientific basis to support this – it's just a guideline. Lots of factors will affect the longevity of a shoe, including how well you look after it, how well it fits, what sort of terrain you run on and your build. It is true that the 'structural integrity' of the shoe will diminish over time but I'd advise going by look and feel rather than the passage of time when deciding whether it's time for a new pair. Rotating different pairs, allowing uppers to dry out and midsoles to decompress between wears, is also likely to extend their life.

To determine whether a shoe is comfortable, you'll need to run in it. A jog around the store won't cut it – you're going to be running in these babies for 26.2 miles (42.2km)! Try to run at least a little way at your goal pace – your stride changes at different speeds and a shoe that feels good at one pace may feel too cumbersome or insubstantial at another. (This offers further support to a study I mention on p. 185 about having multiple shoes 'on the go' at one time, rather than just one pair.) It also raises the question of whether you should have 'racing' shoes.

It's a long-held tradition in running that you have a special pair of shoes to pull out of the bag on race day – traditionally a sleek, more lightweight shoe (often called a racing flat). There could be a psychological benefit to this, I suppose. But for me, that is overridden by the importance of being familiar and comfortable with what I plan to race in. I don't want to get to mile 18 (kilometre 29) and suddenly find I'm getting a blister, or that my calves are screaming in a pair of unfamiliar carbon-plate racing flats. If you do plan to wear race-day shoes, please, please ensure you do at least some of your race-pace training and long runs in them.

## My personal 'right shoe' criteria

When I'm looking for shoes, the three features that would prompt me to put them on my 'try on' pile are weight, shape and heel-toe differential.

In a clever study looking at the effect of shoe weight on performance, researchers sewed lead pellets weighing 100–300g (4–12oz) into the tongues of identical shoes and tested runners in a series of 1.9-mile (3km) time trials. Each 100g (3½oz) of additional weight resulted in a speed that was 1 per cent slower. Weight *does* matter. More to the point though, I just *feel* better in lighter shoes – once they are on, I can forget I'm wearing them.

That's why I'm also picky about fit. Go and get your running shoes and take out the insole. Stand on it, and compare the shape of your foot with the shape of the insole. Your whole foot should be within the boundary of the insole, in order for it to work freely. When the foot lands, the toes should splay to provide stability; when it takes off, the big toe should act as a powerful lever. If the toes are cramped together, these actions can't be performed efficiently.

The heel-toe differential first became a 'thing' when barefoot running and minimalist shoes came to the fore in the late 2000s. After decades of shoes with big padded heels, 'zero drop' shoes, with no difference between the height of the shoe at the heel and the forefoot, became popular. The overall 'stack height' of the shoe – the thickness of the sole – also shrank, allowing runners to feel the ground under their feet more. Since then, the pendulum has swung the other way (with midsole stack heights of up to 40mm/1.6in at the heel) – and someway back again – which at least has left us in a place where there is much more variety on the shelves. I prefer shoes with very little or zero drop. But I would not use that as a reason to recommend them to you. In fact, one study on regular runners found that those wearing shoes with a 10mm (0.4in) drop got injured less than runners wearing a 6mm (0.2in) drop or zero. The takeaway here is that you need to find what works best for you. By all means, take some advice, but ultimately, be guided by your comfort filter.

# Running kit

Enough about shoes. What about kit? You probably already have a wardrobe overflowing with it, so far be it from me to suggest you need more! But here are some considerations for what to wear in different weather conditions.

## Dressing for the heat

If it's going to be a hot day, think about wearing...

### Light colours
Light-coloured clothing absorbs less heat than darker shades.

### Loose-fitting gear
Loose-fitting gear allows more airflow over the skin, which helps sweat evaporate. (It's the evaporation of sweat that cools the body.)

### Less!
Bare skin maximises airflow over the skin to keep you cool. But be wary of sun exposure and protect exposed areas with sunscreen.

### A visor
Keeps the sun off your face, and is preferable to a cap, which will trap heat. The head plays a big role in 'thermal sensation' – our perception of how hot we are as opposed to actual core temperature. A lower thermal sensation can make you feel more comfortable and reduce your RPE.

## Sunglasses

Glare will have you screwing up your face when you're meant to be smiling to stay relaxed and improve your running economy! Sunglasses also protect your eyes from UV rays, grit and flies. Orange, brown or mirrored lenses combat glare and bright light.

## Dressing for the cold

If it's going to be a cold day, think about wearing...

## Layers

Even if it's really chilly, don't make the mistake of opting for a warm, thick top. You want to feel a little cool before you begin running or you'll almost certainly end up too warm. On a cold day, I'll usually opt for a thermal base layer under a T-shirt or vest; if it's slightly less cool, I choose a base layer with a zipped long-sleeve top over the top, which I can undo or remove if I need to.

## Gloves and hat

Keeping your extremities warm makes you feel more comfortable in the cold and these items can usually be stuffed into a pocket or waistband if you get too warm. A cap or visor can be good for keeping rain off your face, especially if you are a glasses wearer.

## Calf sleeves

If you're not ready for tights, calf sleeves (with shorts) can be a good compromise, giving a bit more leg coverage without the risk of overheating (or having soaking wet fabric against your legs). Extra warmth on the calves can help protect against muscle tears, too.

## A waterproof jacket

There's a balance to be struck between breathability and waterproofness. A 'proper' waterproof, with a waterproof coating, taped seams and a hood will be less breathable than a less substantial water-resistant or showerproof jacket. Your choice will be determined by how often you face rainy conditions and how heavy the rain is.

## Carrying fuel

You will almost certainly have to get used to carrying energy gels, drinks or other fuel on your long runs and there are a range of ways to do this, from fuel belts to hydration vests. Consider whether the same method you use in training will work on race day, when the number of gels (or similar) you'll need to carry – and have easy access to – will exceed what you've required in training. One way of finding out is to do a dress rehearsal. The run doesn't need to be particularly long (and obviously, you don't need to consume all those snacks!) but it should be long enough to get a sense of whether your fuel belt, hydration vest or shorts pocket still pass muster. Don't leave this to the last minute, because if you need to explore other options, they too will need to be put to the test before race day.

It isn't necessary to carry your own water in the marathon, unless you really want to, as plenty will be provided on the course. But if you've been using a specific brand of sports drink that you plan to take with you, you'll need to factor that in to your carrying strategy, too.

## Running backpacks

Unless you are taking on a mountain marathon, you're not going to need a backpack for race day. But a running-specific backpack is great to have for destination runs (such as commuting), one-way runs (where you're travelling back on public transport, for example) and even some long runs. You can carry additional clothing, snacks and plenty of fluid as well as essentials like your phone/money.

I have a 17-litre rucksack for when I've got a fair bit to carry and a 10-litre race vest with a hydration bladder for long trail runs and races. Don't carry a bag that's bigger than you need – it's not only extra weight, it's likely to jiggle around more if it's half empty.

# CHOOSING THE RIGHT BAG

### Fit

When testing for fit, adjust the shoulder straps first, then the waist belt and then the chest strap. You need all three for optimal distribution of the weight of the pack, comfort and adjustability. The shoulder and waist straps should be wide enough to provide support without digging in – and adjustable to give a secure fit. A little padding can be nice, but nothing too bulky. The chest strap's main function is to minimise motion. On some models, it is adjustable.

### Size

What do you realistically need to carry? Try putting the things you think you'll be carrying regularly into a few different models to see if they fit well and how the bag feels when it's full. Bags with compression cords are great for securing the contents in a half-full bag.

### Accessibility

Both my rucksacks have front-access pockets. There's nothing more irritating than having to stop to take your bag off in order to get out your phone/lip balm/energy gel. Look for chest compartments with elastic closures and zipped pockets on the waist-belt for valuables.

## Running tech

It's beyond the scope of this book to review the many smart watches, apps and other gadgets out there that can help you record and monitor your running. (And even if I did, the information would be out of date within months!) But as I said in Chapter 4, I advise against relying solely on one single parameter (e.g. pace or heart rate) – make use of the different types of feedback that running tech offers, and always use it in conjunction with – not instead of – how you feel.

# RACING GREEN

Like any mass participation event, a major marathon can have a substantial environmental impact. There's the carbon footprint of runners flying and driving to the race, the mass of plastic water bottles (many of which are discarded with just a few sips taken) and the huge amount of litter, in the form of gel and sweet wrappers and torn bin liners and the mass production of t-shirts, which often end up as bed wear or decorating gear.

Many race organisers are waking up to this problem and taking measures to address it. For example, swapping plastic bottles for disposable cups or offering water fill-ups; reducing the number of water stations, re-using signage, sending out digital race packs instead of paper ones and offsetting their carbon.

There are many ways to reduce your own impact. For example, opt for races closer to home to avoid clocking up air miles. Carry your own water supply or at least, a reusable keep cup, which can be filled at drinks stations. Take your litter away. Trees Not Tees is a company that plants a tree for every runner in a participating event who says 'no thanks' to the race t-shirt (they've planted thousands of trees, across four sites). If the race you're attending isn't signed up, why not suggest it to them? You could also lighten your running wardrobe by donating unwanted gear and kit to worthy causes. Talking of kit, I advise on p. 207 to wear some old, unwanted clothing at the start to keep warm. At major marathons, such as London, Brighton and New York, this clothing is collected up by volunteers for charity. If you're concerned that this won't happen at the race you are running, ask them what will be done with it.

Finally, bear in mind that while there are an increasing number of brands offering apparel and footwear made from recycled or more environmentally friendly materials, the most sustainable kit is the stuff that you already own. Look after it, so that it lasts longer and don't buy what you don't need, be it yet another pair of shorts or the latest smartwatch upgrade.

# BODY MAINTENANCE

# 8

# ROUTINE PROCEDURES

## An in-depth look at warming up, cooling down and the role of flexibility work

I know runners who never warm up, never stretch and never do any activity other than running. Some of them are very successful, rarely troubled by injuries. Others are more like the walking wounded. Equally, I know runners who follow the 'rule book' diligently – yet, once again, while some reap the benefits, others do not. It raises a good question: is it necessary to spend time warming up, cooling down, foam rolling and stretching? Or could you just spend the time running more instead?

## The warm-up

The purpose of a warm-up is to bridge the gap between being at rest and running. When you ease gently into movement, your body temperature increases, heart rate and breathing frequency go up, and blood is directed away from the internal organs to the working muscles. This increase in muscle temperature helps to enhance the efficiency of muscle contractions – one study found that a 1°C (1.8°F) increase was accompanied by a 2–5 per cent improvement in muscle power output.

Articular cartilage, the type that cushions the joints, does not have its own blood supply, relying on nutrients being delivered by a viscous substance called synovial fluid. It is movement that squeezes the synovial fluid into joints, reducing friction between bone surfaces. (That's why far from 'wearing away' joints, running is actually good for them.) So, the benefits of a warm-up are both physiological (gearing up the cardiorespiratory system) and musculoskeletal (mobilising the joints, extending your range of motion and ridding you of unhelpful muscular tension – in other words, peeling those shoulders away from your ears!).

There's a psychological benefit, too: a warm-up encourages you to switch off from the day's worries (be they ahead of you or behind you) and focus on the activity at hand.

Some studies have found a small decrease in the level of post-exercise muscle soreness when a warm-up is performed – but for me, the case for 'making exercise more efficient and comfortable' is a more convincing one than easing post-run aches and pains.

With all this in mind, I am in favour of warming up. Does that mean I spend 15 minutes before every run diligently performing warm-up activities? No.

## Is warming up essential?

There are occasions when a warm-up could be classed as 'useful', and others when it could be classed as 'essential'. If you've been sitting hunched over your computer all day, stuck at the steering wheel or herding a bunch of unruly kids, your body will likely thank you for spending a few moments preparing to run rather than attempting to go from zero to, er, 7mph in one go. If you have particular joints or muscles that tend to feel stiff when you begin running, these are the ones to focus on during your warm-up activities (*see* also 'Ready to roll'). The same goes for if you're recovering from an injury that has left a particular area feeling stiff or tight – often the case with tendinopathies, such as the Achilles or hamstrings.

# READY TO ROLL?

The foam roller is often heralded as a must-have tool for runners – offering a sort of self-administered deep-tissue massage and joint mobilisation through the pressure of your own bodyweight. What does sport science say about the foam roller's benefits? There is reasonable evidence that foam rolling helps to improve joint range of motion prior to exercise, rather like a dynamic warm-up. For example, one study found that combining stretching (static or dynamic) with foam rolling before exercise had an additional positive effect compared to either modality alone (the foam rolling preceded the stretching). Arguably, this just makes the pre-run routine more time-consuming. However, it may be worth experimenting with if you have specific areas that are tight or restricted (such as previously injured sites).

In terms of recovery, where rolling is more commonly used, the science is less compelling. I couldn't find any evidence that it could speed up recovery or attenuate muscle damage. The only area in which it may play a role (other than simple relaxation) is in terms of reducing DOMS after intense exercise.

For those who do roll, the recommendation is to spend 30–120 seconds on each muscle group, rolling in each direction for two to four seconds. Pause on any particularly painful areas, and if possible, shorten and lengthen the muscle that is under pressure by moving the joint (for example, if you find a tight spot on your calf, point and flex your foot). The amount of weight (force) you put through the muscles need not be so much that it makes rolling painful. A study on rolling the quads found that there were no further gains in range of motion when a force eliciting high pain perception was used compared to low and moderate pain perception. So be gentle on yourself.

Finally, avoid rolling directly over the iliotibial band. Not only is it extremely painful but doing so has no benefit at all, since it isn't a muscle. And steer clear of rolling injured tissue while it is healing.

The other crucial consideration in deciding whether and how to warm up is what type of run you're doing. If it's an easy or long run, you might just jog for a few minutes before working up to your desired pace. If possible, I still like to include some mobility exercises (often called 'dynamic stretches'), such as those shown on pp. 136–8, before I ease into the run. For runs that involve greater speed and force output – such as hill training, speedwork or racing – then you will benefit from a more comprehensive warm-up, including mobility exercises, drills (*see* p. 158) or strides (*see* p. 60). Why? Because you'll be taking your joints and muscles through a greater range with faster running, and a more dynamic and specific warm-up will help to prepare them for this.

The timeline on p. 135 shows the 'anatomy' of a running session, from warm-up to cool-down, to help you decide what to include where. But first, let's address the thorny issue of stretching as part of the warm-up.

## Pre-run stretching: the debate goes on

For the last couple of decades, the consensus has been that static stretching (assuming a position in which a muscle is elongated to the point of gentle tension and held for 20–60 seconds) isn't a helpful thing to do before a run.

Indeed, the highly regarded American College of Sports Medicine advises avoiding it within the warm-up routine. This advice is based on research from that period, which found that stretching could reduce the muscles' strength and power output, just when they need to be firing on all cylinders. Neither was any evidence found that stretching before a run decreased post-exercise soreness (DOMS), reduced injury risk or improved performance. This led to the recommendation to save static stretching until after a workout and focus instead on 'dynamic' stretching in the warm-up. (As an example of the difference, a static stretch for the hamstrings might involve raising one leg on to a bench or step and hinging from the hips over that straight leg until you feel a lengthening along the back of the thigh. A dynamic hamstring stretch might entail standing tall while swinging the leg back and forth – so the joint is in motion, rather than held still.)

But recently, there's been some re-examining of this evidence. For one thing, much of that research demonstrating a reduction in muscle power output was based on excessively long 'hold' times. For example, in one meta-analysis reporting a reduction in muscle strength of 5.4 per cent, the average hold time per muscle group was 1½–5 minutes! A more recent study review concluded that while holding stretches for 60 seconds or more *does* have a discernible effect on subsequent strength and power output, stretching for shorter durations – 30–45 seconds per muscle group – has a much less significant impact (the researchers described it as 'insignificant' or 'trivial'). Other recent research suggests that as long as a static stretch is followed up with more dynamic activity, any performance detriment is restored. The type of performance test used to assess the effects of static stretching on subsequent performance has also been challenged. Vertical jump tests or short sprints, which are often used, bear little relevance to endurance running.

All this has led to something of a resurgence of support for static stretching. One recent study concluded 'short-duration static stretching should be included as an important warm-up component before the uptake of recreational sports activities, due to its potential positive effect on flexibility and musculotendinous injury prevention.'

But given that it is recommended as 'part of a comprehensive warm-up routine', which also includes more dynamic movement, it begs the question – why?

Well, maybe so that you don't get injured? A 2016 review found no clear effect of static stretching on all-cause or overuse injuries. It is possible that stretching helps to reduce the risk of muscle and tendon *strain* injuries (the classic hamstring pull or calf tear), which may be of some benefit, but the vast majority of injuries affecting distance runners are overuse, not strain-related (which you can read more about in Chapter 13).

What about static stretching to increase range of motion? Yes, but dynamic stretching can do that too, and is easily incorporated into an active warm-up.

Enhancing performance, then? I've yet to find any evidence that stretching – of any kind – actually makes you run faster. A 2018 study compared the effects of dynamic stretching with static stretching

(3 x 10-second holds) and no stretching. The participants were asked beforehand which option they believed would have the greatest effect on their physical function. The majority chose dynamic stretching – but actually, there were no differences between the groups in terms of physical function or flexibility scores. This ties in with an older study examining the link between stretching and injury. Here, researchers found that when people who customarily stretched were asked not to, they sustained more injuries. A second group, who did not usually stretch but were asked to do so during the study, *also* sustained more injuries. This, perhaps, illustrates that those of us who will benefit from pre-run stretching instinctively do it already. Or that our beliefs have a powerful influence on our actions and their outcomes.

## The verdict

Taking all this research into account, my recommendation on warming up and stretching is this: always warm up before high-intensity running and racing. For other runs, ease in slowly – ideally including some dynamic mobility. If you have plenty of time, or particularly like to do static stretches pre-run, then go for it, but make sure that your muscles are warm before you do so (by preceding them with a few minutes of jogging or other aerobic activity) and follow them with some dynamic activity.

Once you've got a warm-up routine that you feel happy with, stick to it. This becomes a mental trigger that tells your brain: 'We're ready!' It also gives you a game plan for race day when you may feel nervous and end up doing things that you never normally do because you see someone else doing them.

One final thing: don't warm up too long before your session or race begins, otherwise all those fully primed body systems will return to a resting state. This can be particularly challenging at mass-participation marathons, where you are corralled into starting pens early. Read more about race day in Section 5.

# The anatomy of a session

Easy jog – Use the first 5–15 minutes of your run to ease in, gradually increasing pace. Short, fast runs need longer warm-up jogs than long, slow ones. For races, use the last couple of minutes of the warm-up jog to run at your goal pace.

Static stretch – This is not specifically recommended (*see* p. 132) but if you want to stretch before you run, now is the time. Follow up with mobility work, as below.

Mobility work/dynamic stretching – This is recommended before all runs, in an ideal world, but particularly when you've been sedentary/inactive for a long period beforehand and before higher-intensity runs. Many of the moves mentioned on pp. 136–8 can be incorporated into the jog rather than needing to be done separately – this helps to keep your heart rate and body temperature elevated.

Drills – These are recommended before higher-intensity runs such as hills and speedwork. They can also be used as a standalone session or tagged on to an easy run to improve running form. *See* p. 158.

Strides – A useful final transition between the warm-up and any high-intensity workout or race. *See* p. 60.

Session – The run itself.

↓

Cool-down – This involves 5–15 minutes of easy jogging after races, fast-finish runs and high-intensity workouts. Otherwise, it is not essential.

↓

Stretching – It's not necessary to stretch immediately after a run (or at all, some would argue! *See* p. 132). You can stretch at any time – but it can fit well post-run, since your muscles are already nice and warm. Avoid stretching straight after very long runs or races, however.

# MOBILITY EXERCISES

### Leg swings

Stand tall (with support if needed) and swing one leg back and forth. Don't overdo the range. Now swing the leg to the side and across your body. Swap sides.

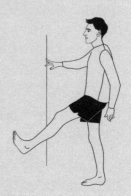

### Walking lunges

Take a big step forwards, allowing the front knee to bend and the rear knee to drop down towards the ground. Drive through the front foot to bring the rear leg up and through into the next step.

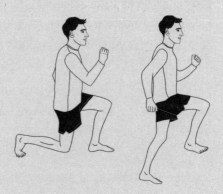

### Hamstring walks

Walking backwards, leave the front foot on the floor, bending the knee of the back leg and flexing at the hips (keep your back straight, not rounded), before stepping backwards with the front foot to adopt the same position on the other side.

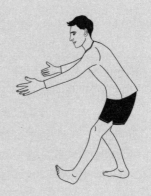

## Knee hugs

Walk forwards, bringing each knee alternately into the chest, momentarily drawing it in with the hands.

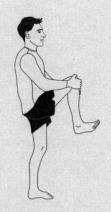

## Heel walking and Toe walking

Walk forwards, with the toes raised and only the heels on the ground. Then lower the toes and raise the heels, to walk on tiptoes.

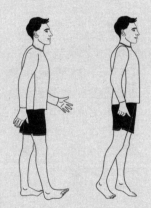

## Hacky sack

Walking forwards, bring your knee up, rotating the knee outwards and the ankle inwards. Tap the ankle with the opposite hand before replacing the foot and repeating on the other leg.

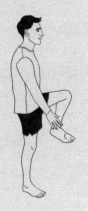

### Crossovers or Carioca

From jogging forwards, turn your body side on and bring the trailing foot across the leading foot on each stride so that you are crossing one over the other. Alternatively, cross the trailing foot in front of the leading foot on one stride and behind it on the next. Remember to change direction.

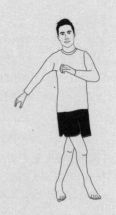

### Sidestepping

From jogging forwards, turn your body side on and step out with the leading leg, bringing the trailing leg in to tap the heels together before stepping out with the leading leg again. Keep your feet pointing directly forwards, not in the direction you are travelling.

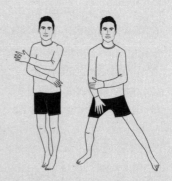

### Heel flicks

From jogging forwards, exaggerate the bend in your knees so that your heels come up towards your bottom. You can do this with one leg at a time (the other leg maintains a normal range of movement) or both at the same time. Keep your arms moving in a running action.

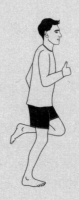

# The cool-down

Cooling down is about transitioning from activity to rest – a warm-up in reverse. The cardiovascular and respiratory systems, as well as neuromuscular function and sweat production, take time to return to a resting state after vigorous exercise, so spending the last few minutes of your run gradually slowing down rather than coming to a sudden and complete stop gives time for this to happen. Just as with the warm-up, the higher the intensity of the workout, the more important this aspect of the session becomes.

Recent research suggests that a cool-down may have another important role. One of the surest determinants of an adaptive response to training is how quickly the 'stress response' can be switched off. This is because repair and adaptation can only take place once the physiological stress of training is no longer present. A faster return to the resting state, then, can enhance adaptation. One study found that an active cool-down (in this case, six minutes of easy cycling) did indeed lead to a more rapid return to a resting state.

Of course, if you don't perform a cool-down, your body will still return to a resting state. Blood lactate, for example, returns to resting levels within 20–120 minutes, even with no active recovery. But the cool-down seems to accelerate the process. Other practices that appear to have a similar effect include listening to music and spending time with fellow runners. Why not combine all three?

In terms of whether a cool-down will hasten your recovery (in other words, whether it'll make you ready to run again sooner) the research is less compelling, although with studies looking at different types of exercise, different durations and different 'markers' of recovery, it's hard to get a clear picture. One study review concluded that a cool-down did not speed recovery or prevent DOMS, but for me, the fact that I feel better for doing one (at least, after high-intensity sessions and races) is enough to negate the need for physiological 'proof' that it is beneficial. A few minutes' jogging gives me a chance to reflect on how the training session went, and to enjoy the feeling of accomplishment before I get on with my day.

## Post-run stretching

And that brings us to stretching. One survey found that almost two-thirds of marathon runners include post-run stretching.

Why do we do it? The most frequently cited reasons include reducing muscle soreness, lowering the risk of injury and maintaining flexibility. As we've already seen, there isn't much evidence that stretching reduces DOMS. A Cochrane Review concluded that the extent to which it reduced soreness the day after exercise was equivalent to one point on a 100-point scale. Nor does stretching offer any protection from overuse injuries, though, as mentioned, it may play a small role in preventing strains.

However, stretching *does* help to increase flexibility when it is performed regularly. Which brings us to an intriguing question – do we want or need more flexibility?

A classic study, back in 2002, found that runners who performed the worst in a 'sit and reach' test (which measures hamstring flexibility) had the best running economy. More recently, it was found that one particular variant (the T variant) of a gene linked to inflexibility, called COL5A1, is found more commonly among runners than non-runners. What's more, runners with the T variant appear to be *faster* than those without it. Researchers believe that a 'stiffer' muscle-tendon unit improves elastic energy storage and return, which increases running efficiency and economy.

But there's a balance to be struck here – between optimal energy return, via muscle-tendon stiffness, and optimal stride length, which demands sufficient range of motion at the hips, knees and ankles. If you are so stiff that taking your limbs through a 'normal' range of motion poses discomfort or risks muscle strain, then I would recommend working on increasing your flexibility. This is particularly important as we age, both for general health and efficient running form. A study from Wake Forest University (2015) comparing runners between 20 and 60 years of age found that stride length was, on average, 20 per cent lower with each decade.

# A fresh approach to stretching

If we take the focus away from stretching being an essential performance-enhancing or injury-preventing strategy and think of it as something that helps us maintain a healthy body with adequate range of motion, it allows us to focus on the specific areas that need addressing, rather than having to follow every run with a full-body stretch (see my recommended 'menu' of stretches over the page.)

It also means that you can separate your stretching time from your running time, if that is easier for you to fit into your routine. For example, you might stretch on your rest days, when you have more time, or after a bath, when your muscles are nicely warm. You might choose to work on flexibility through yoga or Pilates classes. Remember, you're not after gymnast-level range of motion – just an ability to move your joints freely through a healthy range.

Whenever you choose to stretch, do so with good technique and awareness. Don't just go through the motions while scrolling through your phone! Notice if one side is tighter than the other, or if a particular muscle group feels tighter than usual. Take each stretch to a point of mild discomfort – not pain – and hold it for 30 seconds or so (the position, not your breath), ideally performing the stretch more than once.

# YOUR RUNNING STRETCH MENU

### Calves (a)

Take a big step forwards with your right foot, bending the knee. Keep the left leg straight and have both sets of toes pointing directly forwards. Now gently press the heel down into the ground. If you don't feel a stretch, take the left foot further back. To accentuate the stretch, you can also 'grab' the ground with your toes. (If you overpronate when you weight-bear on one leg, rest the big-toe side of your foot on a rolled flannel to prevent it rolling in and letting the calf off the hook.)

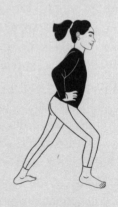

### Calves (b)

Following on directly from the gastrocnemius stretch, take a half-step forwards with your left leg and slightly bend the knee, keeping the left heel on the floor. Look for a stretch along the lower region of the calf. Now repeat both calf stretches on the other side.

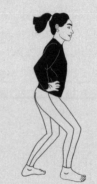

### Hamstrings

Stand in front of a support at mid-shin to mid-thigh height and place your right foot on its surface, with the leg straight. Your support leg should be perpendicular to the ground with the foot facing forwards. Now hinge forwards from the hips until you feel a stretch along the back of the thigh. Don't round or hunch over. If your hamstrings are tight, repeat the stretch with the leg pointing to 1 o'clock and then pointing to 11 o'clock. Finally, perform with the knee slightly bent. You can do the same thing lying down or with your foot on the floor instead of a raised surface.

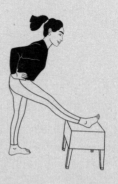

### Hip flexors

Take a large step forwards with your left leg, bending the knee and allowing your right knee to rest on the floor, with the top of your foot facing down. Bring the torso upright and curl your tailbone under to lose your lumbar curve. Then gently press the right hip forwards, squeezing the glute on that leg. Try taking the arm on the side of the stretching leg overhead and flexing to the side. Swap sides.

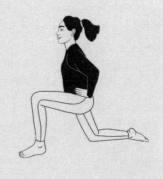

### Quads

Stand tall and take your right foot into your right hand, bringing it towards your bottom. Keep your knees together (don't let the knee of the stretching leg stray out to the side) and keep your torso straight, without arching your back. It doesn't matter if your knee is slightly in front of the supporting leg – this just indicates quad tightness. Swap sides.

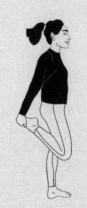

### Mid-back

Begin on all fours, with your hands under your shoulders and your knees under your hips, with your spine neutral (not arched or rounded). Take away your left hand and with your palm upwards, slide it along the floor under your right armpit. Imagine you are trying to get your right shoulder blade stacked on top of your left. Let your head and neck go with you. Keep your hips square to focus the rotation on the thoracic spine. Now repeat on the other side.

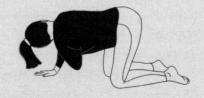

### Hips/glutes (a)

Stand tall and cross your right foot over your left knee. Bend the supporting leg and take the bottom back, as if you were going to sit on an invisible barstool. Gently press the right knee down to stretch the glutes on that side. The alternative is to perform the stretch lying down or seated. Swap sides.

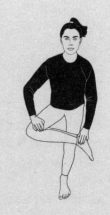

### Hips/glutes (b)

Sit with your right leg extended out on the floor, left leg bent with your foot placed on the outside of your right leg. Wrap your right hand around your left knee and draw it towards you while simultaneously 'resisting' this with your left thigh so that you feel a stretch in the left hip and a rotation in the spine.

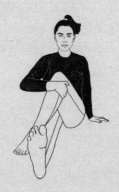

### Inner thighs

Stand with your feet wider than hip-width apart, toes pointing directly forwards on both feet. Now shift your weight over the right foot, keeping the torso upright and bending the right knee. Keep your left foot anchored and the leg straight. Feel a stretch along the inner border of the left leg. Swap sides.

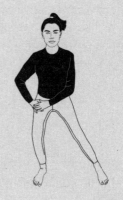

# 9

# RAPID RECOVERY

## The role of rest and recovery – and how to make it count

You can't 'force' recovery from a hard run or race. It takes time. But there are a few things that can help or hinder the process. Before we take a closer look at these, I want to highlight a fascinating study conducted back in 2014, which demonstrates just how much our beliefs influence what we experience.

Researchers from Victoria University in Australia told one group of participants that the lukewarm water they were about to immerse their limbs in, post-workout, contained a special 'recovery oil'. Another group were assigned plain warm water and a third group, cold water. The results? Recovery – gauged by pain levels, leg strength and readiness to exercise again – was significantly quicker among the 'recovery oil' group compared to the warm water group and equal to those who bathed in cold water.

The scientific evidence on many commonly recommended recovery practices is equivocal. That doesn't mean you shouldn't try them. But it does mean that what works for one may not for another, and that your belief or disbelief in any particular practice can strongly influence the outcome.

# Refuel

One practice that doesn't raise any such controversy is post-run refuelling and hydration. You can read more about the key components of refuelling in detail on pp. 231–3, but suffice it to say here that taking in some carbohydrate and protein within an hour of your workout is the most important step you can take in kick-starting recovery (and ideally, a pre-bedtime hit of protein, too). Don't wait until you've checked your stats on Strava and had a shower!

# Chill out

Talking of showers, what about the proverbial ice bath? Cryotherapy – be it an ice bath, a bag of frozen peas on your sore knee or a session in a cryochamber (where you are exposed to extremely low-temperature vapours for a short period) – has become a widespread recovery tool in many sports. But it's a tricky subject. While it isn't refuted that cryotherapy has a dampening effect on many of the biomarkers associated with inflammation and damage – including a reduction in DOMS – some scientists question whether this is actually a good thing. It's argued that many aspects of this inflammatory response play an important role in triggering exercise-induced adaptations and that preventing it through cryotherapy (or indeed, other anti-inflammatory practices) could ultimately attenuate the long-term adaptive response to training. In one study, volunteers exercised for four to six weeks, with sessions followed either by cold-water immersion (CWI) or no treatment. Training effects (assessed by parameters of muscular performance) were three times greater in the group whose muscles were *not* cooled after training.

Other studies simply question whether cryotherapy works. A 2018 randomised controlled trial on post-marathon recovery concluded 'cryotherapy is no more effective than a placebo intervention at improving functional recovery or perceptions of training stress following a marathon.'

Another 2018 study looked at the effects of cooling, warming and no treatment on the recovery of fatigued legs following endurance exercise. They found that *warming* the muscles improved muscle function more successfully than did cooling – and that the cooling treatment hampered glycogen resynthesis (the replenishment of glycogen within the muscles and liver). However, critics say that the extremely long heating/cooling period – two hours – that the study used does not mimic 'real life', where cold-water immersion is more likely to last 10–15 minutes. They cite research showing that this more realistic duration of cold-water immersion has no negative effect on glycogen resynthesis.

One question to ask yourself when deciding whether or not to take the plunge is what is your motivation? If you are doing it because you think it will make you a better athlete, then you might want to reconsider. If you're doing it because you think it will make you *feel* better, then go ahead.

Should you fork out for a pricey cryotherapy chamber session? Interestingly, plain old cold-water immersion fares better in the research. Studies suggest that the hydrostatic pressure is one likely factor, but the lowering of core body temperature and muscle temperature is also thought to repair muscle damage, attenuate strength loss and ease feelings of fatigue. The best protocol is to swiftly get into water of 10–13°C (50–55.4°F) following exercise, immerse as much of your body as you can and stay there for 10 minutes. But if the prospect of doing so fills you with dread, you now have some justification to opt for a warm shower instead.

I'll talk more about applying ice topically to specific sore areas on p. 190.

## Get some shut-eye

Eliud Kipchoge reportedly naps for two hours each day. Paula Radcliffe slept 10 hours a night when she was an elite marathon runner. Sleep is a crucial part of your running lifestyle – just as important as good nutrition. And yet it's something so many of us still neglect. A study in 2019 showed that endurance athletes who got less than seven hours a night were more likely to succumb to injury over the course of a year than those who got more than seven hours.

While there is no set amount of sleep that is ideal for every individual, it's certainly true that not getting enough shut-eye has many negative consequences for running – increased RPE during exercise, a compromised immune system, poor decision making, slower muscle recovery and repair, and higher pain perception.

One of the reasons that sleep is so important from a recovery point of view relates to growth hormone (GH). This hormone, released by the pituitary gland, plays a key role in growth and regeneration (read: adaptation to exercise) – especially the repair and renewal of muscle tissue and bone and the enhancement of fat metabolism. Exercise (particularly above the lactate threshold) stimulates the release of GH, but the highest levels of secretion take place during sleep and it's been shown that not getting enough can lead to growth hormone resistance (in other words, the adaptations and repair work that would normally happen are compromised). Incidentally, a high level of alcohol consumption also decreases GH secretion.

Recently, there has been some research looking at the idea of 'banking' sleep. This means intentionally sleeping more prior to a period when you are likely to be sleep-deprived. The obvious scenario in which this could be of great value to a marathon runner is the night before the race, when many of us end up staring at the ceiling, wide eyed. A study on basketball players found that aiming for 10 hours a night minimum for five to seven weeks (if only!) had a positive effect on many aspects of their game, but research specifically looking at endurance performance found that additional sleep (in the form of a nap) only influenced time to exhaustion in runners who were already sleep-deprived, and not those who were well rested.

If you struggle to get up in the mornings or frequently feel exhausted during the day, consider finding a way to increase your sleep hours, regardless of whether you already get seven or eight hours a night or not. It might mean going to bed earlier, grabbing daytime naps or improving your sleep 'hygiene' so that you get to sleep more quickly and enjoy more uninterrupted sleep. I often sneak in an afternoon nap after long runs and races. Turning off my phone an hour or so before bed has also worked wonders for me, whether that is to do with the screen's blue light or the fact that I don't go to bed worrying about emails or gloomy news stories I've just read.

## Ease sore muscles

I do not routinely stretch after a long or hard run. When muscles feel tender, it's because they have undergone microscopic damage (microtrauma) and the inflammatory response has set in to protect them. It's not wise, therefore, to stress them further through stretching. Leave it till later, or a different day, when they feel better. The same goes for foam rolling (which you can read more about on p. 131). However don't just glue yourself to the sofa for the rest of the day, either. Gentle movement – like walking, or gentle swimming – promotes blood flow and can stop you feeling so stiff.

## The big squeeze

I often put on compression tights or calf sleeves following a long run. One study found that donning a pair of knee-high compression socks for 48 hours after a marathon had a positive effect on recovery. (Recovery was demonstrated by a 2.4 per cent improvement in time to exhaustion on a treadmill run two weeks after the marathon, compared to a 3.6 per cent *decline* in those who did not wear the socks.)

Other recent research on cyclists found that perceived muscle soreness following a fatiguing bout of cycling was lower after wearing compression tights for 60 minutes compared to a control group. The tights-wearing cyclists also performed better in a subsequent 'all-out' cycling test. However, another recent study could not find any reduction in DOMS when compression socks were worn during – and for six hours after – exercise.

I definitely would not claim the science supporting compression for recovery is resounding, but there is enough evidence to suggest they can at least make you *feel* better (seen in a lower level of perceived exertion or pain rating), which in itself may have a positive impact on recovery.

## There's the rub

A sports massage therapist is a key part of the team surrounding most elite athletes. And yet the scientific evidence supporting its efficacy is surprisingly scant. A 2016 evidence review concluded the effects of massage on recovery were 'rather small and partly unclear' although the same year, a Brazilian study found that a seven-minute post-event massage significantly reduced subjective pain and fatigue scores in a group of Ironman triathletes. A more recent study review (2021) concluded that while there was no evidence of improvement in measures of performance (including strength, endurance, sprint speed or jump height) following massage, there was some evidence that it could slightly reduce DOMS and improve post-run flexibility.

It appears that rather than flushing out toxins, the benefits of massage come from the pressure it exerts on muscles and other connective tissue – an action known as mechanotherapy.

Despite these mixed findings, I won't be giving up my semi-regular sports massages. I see it as a reward for all my hard work, for one thing. And once the therapist gets to know your body, it can also serve as an early-warning system, highlighting uncommon tightness or tenderness that may hint of a forthcoming problem.

## Make the most of your rest days

One final thing to consider when it comes to optimising recovery is what you do on your rest days. Non-running days should not be physically taxing. This is not the time to get on with your house renovation project, spend the day on your feet or, heaven forbid! go on a huge bender... Nor should you wear yourself out with other physical activities (see Chapter 2 for a reminder of the role of cross-training in your marathon programme). The more frequently you run, the more crucial this point is. For example, if you only run three or four days a week, you have quite a few rest days to play with – but if you run five or six days a week then you need to be more disciplined about how you spend them, so that you don't return to training in an under-recovered state.

That isn't to say that you must be completely and fully recovered before you train again – dealing with 'accumulated fatigue' is all part of the training process. But being overly fatigued is likely to dent your fitness gains either by overloading an already stressed body or by reducing the effort that you are able to put into the next session. Following a well-structured training plan will avoid this as long as you also stay tuned to your own body and honour your instincts.

# 10
# RUN BETTER

## Improving your running skill

Watching a runner with good technique is like poetry in motion. Their movement is strong and purposeful, yet fluid and relaxed. It's also economical, both in the sense that they don't squander energy on unnecessary movement or poor control – and in terms of how much oxygen they use to fuel their efforts. One study found that elite male distance runners used 6 per cent less oxygen at a fixed pace than did recreational runners, and their more efficient running form undoubtedly plays a role in this.

Running is a skill. That's not to say you can't do it *without* skill, but through attention and practice, you can improve the way you run, just as with attention and practice you can improve the way you swim front crawl or swing a golf club. Whatever your current running form, it is unlikely that it's entirely 'good' or 'bad' – which means there's always something to improve! That's why even the elites spend time working to improve their technique, when to the casual observer they may already appear textbook perfect. Like them, I believe that any degree of improvement can pay dividends.

## Why do we run badly?

There are a number of different reasons why we don't run as well as we could. Some running form 'inefficiencies' – such as looking down at your feet – are simply bad habits or down to a lack of awareness of what you're doing. That's why watching a video clip of yourself running can be so revelatory – surely that's not *you* shuffling along with your right shoulder up by your ear?!

Getting someone to record you on your phone (slow-motion is particularly useful) or asking those who regularly run with you what your 'characteristic' form foibles are can be really helpful. (Apparently, I can be recognised from the back by the way my right foot turns out to 1 o'clock!) While external feedback is useful, it's also important to hone your ability to tune into the feedback your body is giving you. *See* 'Seven ways to run better' on the next page.

A common cause of biomechanical faults – such as your feet crossing over an imaginary midline (known as a 'crossover gait') or poor hip extension – is a lack of the necessary strength, mobility or movement skill (co-ordination, balance or proprioception, for example) to accomplish the required action. Even when we start out running with relatively good form, faults can creep in as we become more fatigued. We sit in the hips more (so the bottom sticks out), hunch forwards or shuffle. I'm a big proponent of regular strength and conditioning work to combat this. *See* Chapter 11 to find out more.

A final factor in poor running technique is a misunderstanding of what we 'should' be doing. For example, some runners kick their feet up high towards their bottoms when they run, because they've observed that fast runners' feet do this and concluded that it must be 'correct'. But the reason a fast runner's feet come up so high is because of the high force they've exerted against the ground. Their feet have effectively 'bounced' up. So *pulling* them up, using muscular effort, isn't the same thing at all. Other runners move their arms backwards and forwards in a straight line, like robots, rather than allowing the arms to follow the natural rotation of the body. (Watch Eliud Kipchoge and the team of runners who accompanied him on his world-breaking sub-2-hr-marathon if you need convincing about this.)

## Should you change your form?

To improve, then, you first need to know what actually constitutes good running form. Then you need to know what you are currently doing, and what can be tweaked or improved upon. The final stage is determining how best to implement those changes. All this means that working on your running form takes time and energy – it may even require you to run less, while you focus on the *quality* of your movement.

If you're about to begin your marathon build-up, then this is probably not the best time to be making large-scale changes to the way you run. However, if you feel that your current running form is holding you back, or leading to frequent or recurring injuries, then establishing a better movement pattern before you begin increasing your training volume for the marathon (or certainly no later than the Foundation phase of your marathon-training programme) might be appropriate. I'd recommend working with a good coach or biomechanics expert to do this.

Ask yourself the following questions to help you decide whether you need to make changes:

☑ Do I suffer from lots of injury problems?
☑ Have specific faults in my technique been identified?
☑ Am I willing to put in the time and effort to change my running technique?
☑ Is having 'good form' important to me?

Even if now isn't the right time for a full-on focus on running form – or if you're in the 'if it ain't broke, don't fix it' camp – there are some tweaks, cues and self-checks that can help you run more comfortably and efficiently without needing to 'rebuild' from the ground up. Having a toolbox of techniques to draw on when running is feeling difficult (such as when you're struggling late on in a race) can be really valuable.

## Seven ways to run better

1. Relax. It's much harder to run efficiently if you are tense. Eliud Kipchoge deliberately uses smiling as a tool to send 'relax' signals to his body as he gets tired and maintaining pace gets harder – and science backs him up. Research in the journal *Psychology of*

*Sport and Exercise* found that smiling improves running economy and lowers rate of perceived exertion, while frowning does the opposite. Be aware of other common tension sites, including the hands (unclench those fists and relax your thumbs) and the shoulders.

2. Run tall. You might want to imagine a helium balloon is pulling you upwards from the crown of your head, but the feeling should be subtle and should not create any sense of effort or tension. A very slight forward lean (think of it from the ankles to the ears) is fine – one study found that the average lean among a group of elite runners was 3.5 degrees – but do not bend forwards from the waist. It can help to think of the logo on your running top pointing forwards not down to the ground.

3. Avoid overstriding. When the foot lands too far out in front of you, it has to stay on the ground longer, 'waiting' for your body to travel over the leg before it can come off the ground. This increases your ground contact time, slowing the gait cycle down. It also means you lose out on that free elastic energy stored in your muscles and tendons, and need to use more muscular effort to get off the ground. Overstriding tends to result in landing with a straighter leg, which increases the stress going through the joints, particularly the knee. Shortening stride by 10 per cent reduced the risk of shin injuries by 3–6 per cent in one study.

4. Have fast feet. Cadence is the speed at which the feet turn over, measured in steps per minute. Efficient runners tend to have a relatively high cadence; they pick up their feet quickly, which greatly reduces overstriding and enables them to utilise more elastic energy. There is no magical cadence for which all runners should aim (including the oft-cited 180spm) – cadence is influenced by many things; height and leg length but more importantly, pace. (Running faster makes your cadence go up.) That said, there is definitely evidence that a slow, 'sticky' cadence is inefficient. A cadence of 160spm or less would generally qualify as slow. One recent study from the University of Wisconsin-La Crosse found that increasing cadence by 10 per cent reduced average peak impact force by 5.6 per cent while another found increasing cadence by 7.5 per cent reduced forces on the knee joint. *See* 'What's your cadence?' for advice on assessing and improving your cadence.

## WHAT'S YOUR CADENCE?

Many smart watches monitor cadence – which you can view as an average across the whole run or by 'lap'. Make sure you assess yourself on flat, even terrain and try to run at your usual 'comfortable run' pace. No device? No problem. Simply count the number of steps you take with one foot over one minute of steady-paced running – multiply this by two to get your current cadence. If there's room for improvement (if your cadence is around 160spm or lower), aim for an increase of around 5–8 per cent. A metronome (available as a clip-on device or phone app) can be set to this new tempo to give you a rhythm to follow (a metronome was used in the University of Wisconsin-La Crosse study mentioned on p. 154). I advise using a metronome over a short period only – say, the first five minutes of a run – or even just as a warm-up activity, to help ingrain the 'new' cadence into your mind before you set off. It can also be useful for drills and strides.

5. Be fully armed. The arm action in running counterbalances the movement of the legs as well as helping to propel you at faster speeds. In order to help and not hinder, your arms should be bent to at least 90 degrees (a shorter 'lever' can move more quickly than a longer one) and you should maintain this elbow bend throughout the arm swing, rather than reaching forwards with the hands on the forward swing or 'flinging' the forearm back during the back swing. Allow your forearms to travel towards the midline as they come forwards (following the curve of the ribcage) – and remember that as your torso rotates slightly on each stride, the midline shifts with it. Now drop your shoulders.

6. Look forward. Your head weighs approximately 3–5kg (6.6–11lb) depending on how brainy you are(!), so be smart and look a few metres ahead, not down, otherwise the weight of it will pull your torso forwards, wrecking your tall posture.

7. Body scan. 'Body scanning' is a great way of monitoring your form while you run. Imagine you have an X-ray machine and make a 'virtual tour' of your entire body from head to toe, looking for energy wasters like tight shoulders, clenched fists, a heavy foot strike or slumped posture. A regular check-in, perhaps every mile, or each time you take a drink, helps you remain attentive to any obvious faults that you can address to make running feel more comfortable and fluid.

## Should I worry about foot strike?

There is still much debate about the relative merits of 'forefoot striking' and 'heel striking'. It's often inferred that heel striking is 'bad' or 'novice' and forefoot striking is 'good' and 'expert', with studies showing that while the vast majority of recreational runners land heel first, forefoot striking is more common among faster runners. My observation is that efficient runners often *do* forefoot strike (or land with the foot fairly flat, sometimes called 'midfoot striking'), but the more important issue is *where* the foot lands in relation to your body. A strong heel strike (i.e. landing on the rear of the heel with the ankle very flexed) is often associated with overstriding (see above) and it is this that is the technique problem, rather than the heel landing per se. I've noticed that some elite runners land with a subtle heel strike but still with their foot touching down below, not ahead of, the knee. Conversely, I've seen runners landing on the balls of their feet – probably believing they are running efficiently – who are still extending their legs way out in front of them (giving a rather balletic look), putting undue stress on the foot musculature and bones.

Research from the University of Delaware has shown that a heel strike induces loads that are more associated with tibial stress fractures (shin splints), while a forefoot strike is associated with mechanics that place a runner at greater risk for Achilles tendonitis. This suggests that rather than being associated with a higher or lower injury risk, different foot strike patterns are simply associated with *different* injury risks.

With increased awareness and drills to reduce overstriding and develop a good cadence, you will almost certainly improve the position of your landing foot – and you may find that you move further away from a heel strike. I think this is a better way of approaching things than putting the focus entirely on 'trying' to avoid a heel strike or intentionally switching to a forefoot strike.

# Running cues

A 'cue' is an instruction aimed at giving you an idea of how a movement should feel. For example, 'run tall' or 'lean from the ankles'. Cues can be incredibly helpful, but can also be a bit hit and miss, because what resonates with one runner can be misinterpreted – or meaningless – to another (as I've found through my own coaching!).

Here are my favourite three cues. Try implementing them, one a time, over 50m (55 yards) or so. They might help. But if they don't, leave them out of your toolbox.

## 1. Lead with the knee

The visualisation here is that your knee comes forwards ahead of your foot, so that when it lands, your shin is roughly vertical. This helps to prevent overstriding and eliminate a heel strike. However, don't confuse leading with the knee with 'knees up', which results in unnecessary and unhelpful effort.

## 2. Fast and light

This refers not to your running speed, but specifically to the rhythm of your feet. It encourages a high cadence and a light, nimble foot strike that is more like kissing the ground with your foot than stomping over it.

## 3. Push the ground behind you

When your knee is up and forward, think 'down and back', as if you're going to push the ground away with your foot as it makes contact. Imagine you are riding a scooter and how you would have to push the ground away and extend your leg behind you to propel yourself forwards. This cue helps to improve hip extension.

# Running drills

While a cue provides something to focus on during normal running, a drill extracts a specific aspect of running form to work on in isolation. The idea is that by working on individual elements independently, when you put it all back together, you end up with a more polished stride. Drills also build running-specific strength and movement skill. Here are three to try...

## 1. A–skip

This is a bit like the sort of travelling skip a child would do, but with a shorter stride length and a more rapid rhythm. Each knee is raised alternately – so that the raised heel is level with the supporting leg's knee. As the foot drops directly down, it performs a small hop while the other knee springs up. Make sure you don't reach out with the foot or land on the heel. The arms are used in a running action. The aim is to improve foot placement and optimise the use of elastic energy. It can also be used to promote a faster cadence. Perform the drill twice over 15–20m (16–22 yards).

## 2. Straight–leg running

This drill improves recruitment of the glutes and hamstrings just before and at foot strike, and encourages you to land beneath yourself. Run forwards at a slow pace with your legs completely straight. Maintain a tall posture and do not lean back. Focus on the 'pulling back' of the leg, rather than seeing it as a 'kicking forward' movement. Use your arms in a running action and land on the ball of the foot. You should feel springy. Perform twice over 15–20m (16–22 yards).

## 3. Controlled bounding

This drill helps to enhance hip extension power and elastic energy return. Run forwards at a slow pace and try to increase the amount of time you spend in the air by driving off the ground with more force than usual and using a vigorous arm action. You should feel as if you momentarily 'hang' in the air with each stride before landing on the ball of the foot. Perform two rounds of 8–12 bounds.

## Take a breath

There are lots of theories on the best way to breathe during running – belly breathing, specific rhythms entrained (synchronised) to your foot strike, nasal breathing, in through the nose, out through the nose... There are even whole books on it. If you feel that your breathing is something that holds your running back, you could delve into the subject. You might also want to check in with your doctor to rule out any breathing-related issues such as exercise-induced asthma.

But honestly? Breathing is a natural process to get oxygen into the body and since you are running, you want as much of that as possible, so anything that restricts it (such as nasal breathing, or having to concentrate on breathing in for a certain number of counts and out for a different number of counts) is likely to have a detrimental effect. The mouth is a far bigger airway than the nose, which is why trying to breathe only through your nose isn't a good idea. Sure, you might *also* breathe through your nose (called 'oronasal breathing') but as an adjunct, not a substitute.

The theory behind the claim that an uneven inhale-exhale pattern (inhaling for three steps, exhaling for two, for example) is better than an even one (inhaling for two steps, exhaling for two) is that the body is less able to withstand the impact of landing during an exhale compared to an inhale. So if you always breathe out when, say, your right foot is landing, you are more likely to get an injury than if you spread the load by alternating your exhale from right foot strike to left foot strike. This finding is often attributed to a study that observed breathing patterns during running. The study hypothesised that humans co-ordinate breathing and locomotion to reduce the energy cost of the breathing muscles and to minimise unhelpful mechanical interactions between body parts involved in breathing and running. But the authors stress that while some runners display a 2:1 breathing pattern and others a 3:1 pattern, many have no discernible pattern at all – and even within individuals, breathing patterns can be variable. They also don't link a reduced injury risk or improved performance to switching to an uneven pattern.

In my opinion, the best way to breathe is the way that feels most natural to you. You will be more aware of your breathing when you are running hard compared to on easy runs, and if you feel out of breath on easy runs, it's a sign that you are going too fast. I will offer just two pieces of advice on breathing. First, don't hold your tummy in. It's fine to have your abdominals gently engaged, but pulling your belly button back to your spine locks your ribcage and diaphragm, restricting your breathing capacity (try it). Second, if you feel you can't get enough breath in, focus on breathing out. At the end of an outbreath, inhalation happens automatically. Just for the record, running coach Jack Daniels observes that over 80 per cent of elite marathon runners use a 2:2 breathing pattern.

# 11

# BE A STRONGER RUNNER

## How strength and conditioning can raise your running game

High mileage and long distances take their toll on the body. Building your training up gradually – and scheduling in recovery time – go some way to helping your body withstand the stresses on the musculoskeletal system. But for my money, strength and conditioning (S&C) are key.

Strength and conditioning are often lumped together, or the words used interchangeably – but there is a difference. Strength training is aimed specifically at improving your muscles' capacity to exert (or resist) a force, while conditioning is a broader umbrella; referring to exercises or activities that maintain or improve your ability to run well – such as balance and stability, co-ordination, posture and mobility – without necessarily enhancing your force output.

### May the force be with you

You might not think of running as being about force. It's not as if you carry weights with you, or try to leap as high as possible into the air. But how fast you run is directly related to how much force you can produce against the ground on each stride. And because strength training demands a lot from the muscles, it promotes the recruitment of more muscle fibres, which can then step in when the going gets tough during runs, spreading the workload more widely and helping you resist fatigue.

While both strength and conditioning are important, a good level of conditioning is a *prerequisite* for strength training. Even if you have the strongest, most powerful hip extensors to propel yourself forwards with, if you can't stabilise at the pelvis and knee on landing, you won't be able to make best use of that strength in terms of stride efficiency – and you'll be at greater risk of injury.

The Foundation Plan on p. 164 provides a good introduction to strength and conditioning for anyone who isn't currently doing any. You can start this plan at any time, or follow it during the Foundation phase of one of the marathon programmes in this book.

## A question of load

To elevate your running performance, though, you'll need to bring in the heavies. A detailed analysis of 24 studies published in the journal *Sports Medicine* (2017) showed that resistance training with weights boosted running economy by 2–8 per cent and time trial or race performance in endurance events by 2–4 per cent. Maximal sprint speed also increased. Compound exercises (those that use multiple muscle groups simultaneously) such as squats, deadlifts, lunges and step-ups were the most commonly prescribed exercises.

Is it really necessary to load up with weights? Given that running entails contracting muscles over and over, against low resistance, instinct might lead you to think that lots of repetitions with a relatively light weight would be the way to go – especially since runners don't want to be weighed down with bulky muscle.

Sure, if you've never done any strength training, light weights will make a difference initially, but research shows that it is not the best way to make performance gains in running. Heavy resistance training (along with explosive strength training and plyometrics) is more effective because it gets more muscle fibres recruited – not just the slow-twitch ones that are recruited at low intensity.

The Performance Plan on p. 169 focuses on building strength specifically related to running. That doesn't mean every exercise will 'look' like running. For example, some are double-leg movements, even though you are never on both feet at the same time during the running stride. In these cases, the direction and rate at which force is exerted are what's relevant, even though the movement itself doesn't resemble running.

The goal with this plan, as the name suggests, is to improve running performance, rather than provide a general body workout or reduce injury risk. If you are already comfortable with strength and conditioning work, you can start this plan straight away, or within the Foundation phase of your marathon programme. But don't be tempted to go straight to the Performance Plan if you aren't already doing any regular strength and conditioning. Build your foundation first.

## Perfecting posture

Regardless of which plan you choose, it is essential to do the exercises with good posture. Whenever I mention posture, I notice people pin back their shoulders and stick out their chests! Good posture, though, isn't about creating tension – quite the opposite. When the skeleton is properly aligned, the muscles actually have to do less work to maintain posture.

- ☑ Start by standing tall. Think of a helium balloon drawing you upwards, so that the back of your neck is long.
- ☑ Let your shoulders fall away from your ears, the shoulder blades dropping down your back. Your sternum (the bone in the centre of your chest) faces forwards, not down towards the ground in front. Your tummy can be gently 'engaged' or drawn in, but don't pull it in tightly or you'll restrict your breathing and prevent your torso from rotating. Your back should be neither overly arched nor flexed: take hold of the sides of your pelvis and try tilting it forwards (so your back arches) and backwards (so the back flattens) to find a comfortable midpoint.
- ☑ From a sideways view, the shoulder, hip and ankle should be 'stacked' on top of one another, the knee straight but not pushed back.
- ☑ The weight under your feet should feel equally distributed between left and right – and under each foot, on three points of a tripod: the ball of the big toe, the ball of the little toe and the heel. And breathe!

# FOUNDATION PLAN

Do the exercises below with good posture, focus and control. You can do them whenever suits you best, on rest days or run days, though ideally avoid doing them when you are fatigued and may not be able to maintain good technique. Aim for two to three workouts per week for eight weeks. After that once a week is enough to maintain what you've gained – or you could move on to the Performance Plan on p. 169.

## Goblet squat

*hip and thigh strength, ankle flexibility, adductor length*

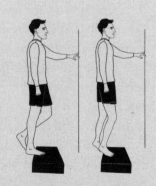

Stand with your feet a little wider than your hips, feet pointing slightly outwards and hands clasped at the front of your chest (holding a light weight if you wish). Initiate the squat by flexing at the hips as if to sit down on something behind you, allowing the thighs to reach roughly parallel with the ground (less far if you are unable to do this without rounding or arching the back or if it hurts your knees). Keep your chest up (your torso and shins should be approximately aligned with each other) and ensure your knees track over your middle toes. If they tend to roll in, brace them outwards, or use a resistance band around your lower thighs to push out against.
PERFORM 3 X 10–15 REPS.

## Functional calf raises

*calf and ankle strength, stability and mobility*

Stand tall holding on to a support with just the front half of your right foot on a step, the other leg dangling freely. Drop the right heel down below the level of the step, bending the knee at the same time. Now lift the heel, but only straighten the knee at the top of the movement. Lower with a straight knee to return to the start position for the next rep.

If you have heel or Achilles issues, perform this movement from a flat surface instead of a step. (i.e. bend the knee, extend through the ankle, then straighten the knee at the top of the movement.)
PERFORM 2–3 X 10–25 REPS PER LEG. YOU SHOULD BE ABLE TO MANAGE 25 REPS BEFORE ADDING WEIGHT

## Single-leg dips
*hip-knee alignment, eccentric quad strength, ankle flexibility*

Stand on one leg with the lifted knee bent, your foot roughly in line with the standing-leg shin. Cross your hands over your chest. Bend the standing-leg knee, keeping the pelvis level, the knee aligned over the middle toe and the torso upright. (This is NOT a squatting movement.) If necessary, hold a support to maintain balance and alignment. Pause in the bent-knee position, then straighten the leg fully. To make it more challenging, loop a resistance band just below the standing-leg knee and secure it to something across your body. This will pull your knee inwards, recruiting the lateral glutes and tibialis posterior (a lower leg muscle that helps control the foot) to resist this movement.
PERFORM 2–3 X 10–12 REPS PER LEG.

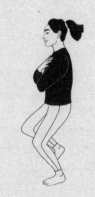

## Forward lunge
*eccentric quad strength, pelvic stability, control of landing*

Standing tall with your feet hip-distance apart, step forwards into a lunge, bending your front knee and taking the back knee towards the ground. Keep your torso aligned over your hips. Pause, then drive back up through the front foot to standing. Now lunge on the other leg. Don't lunge so far that your knee ends up ahead of your foot. Imagine there is a white line running from the midline of your body and on to the floor, and ensure that you step either side of the line rather than across it.

If you tend to hunch or lean forwards in running, then try bringing your arms overhead on the lunge, returning them to your sides on the way back up.
PERFORM 3 X 12–16 ALTERNATE REPS.

### Glute bridge

*strengthen glutes and hamstrings*

Lie on your back with your knees bent to around 45 degrees, feet on the floor and arms across your chest or on the floor. Raise your pelvis without arching your back, hold for five seconds, then lower and repeat (a). Placing your feet further away from your bottom focuses more on the upper hamstrings; having your feet closer to your bottom focuses on the glutes. If the exercise feels very easy with two feet on the ground, progress to single-leg bridges (b): from the lifted pelvis position, alternately lift each foot a few inches, keeping the knee bent. Make sure you are able to keep the pelvis level and stable as you do this. Switch legs between sets.

PERFORM 2–3 X 8–12 HOLDS OR ALTERNATE REPS.

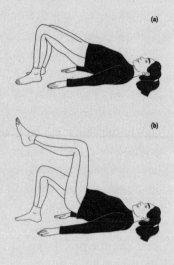

### Heel touchdowns

*control of neutral spine, anti-extension*

Lying on your back with your spine in a neutral position, draw both knees up so that your hips and knees are bent to 90 degrees (a). Draw in your belly button, lightly tensing the lower abdomen. Lower one foot to tap the ground with the heel, (b) maintaining your spinal curves and using the abdominals to control the leg's descent (the back should not arch or flatten during the movement). Draw the leg back up and lower the other heel. When you can do this with control, extend the leg straight as it lowers.

PERFORM 3 X 10–12 REPS.

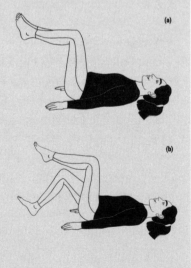

## Back extension
*postural control, thoracic mobility*

Lie face down (a) with your arms bent by your sides (your hands should be on the ground, between your shoulders and forehead, forearms a little away from, but parallel to, your torso). Let the pelvis stay heavy on the floor and rise up on to your forearms, visualising your breastbone reaching forwards and feeling your spine extend (b). Don't hunch your shoulders. Pause, then 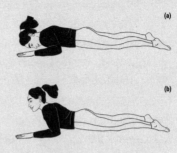 slowly lower. If this feels easy, you can momentarily lift the forearms off the ground in the extended position before replacing them to roll back down through the spine. Ensure that your shoulder blades are drawing down your back and that you extend through the whole spine, not just the lower back. PERFORM 2–3 X 8–12 REPS.

## Side plank
*trunk strength, postural control, anti-extension*

The side plank is my favourite trunk exercise – it's more relevant to running than a front plank as it challenges the gluteus medius, an important hip stabiliser. Lie on one side with your elbow below your shoulder and your top leg stacked on top of your bottom leg. 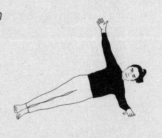 Lift the side of your waist up away from the floor to form a straight line with your body. Don't arch your back. Raise your top arm vertically, keeping your head aligned with your body. Breathe! Swap sides. PERFORM 1–3 REPS PER SIDE, HOLDING FOR UP TO 30 SECONDS.

To progress, try holding a light weight in the raised hand and rotating it to challenge stability, or raising the top leg without letting your body sink towards the floor. If the side plank is too challenging, dial it back by bending the bottom leg and keeping the knee on the floor.

You can alternate the side plank with a prone (front) plank, making sure that you begin with your elbows under your shoulders, shoulder blades drawn down the back and your body in a straight line, with no sagging or humping.

### Resisted foot inversion

*intrinsic foot strength and mobility, control of pronation*

The tibialis posterior muscle sits deep within the calf, crossing the ankle to insert underneath the foot. It is essential to the control of impact and pronation and is a big player in the prevention of plantar fasciitis. Sit on a chair and cross your left foot over the top of the right, tucking it next to it. Hook a resistance band around the ball of your left foot, with the other end secured somewhere to your left. Keeping your left heel anchored, draw the ball of the foot away to the right in an arcing motion, keeping the knees pressed together

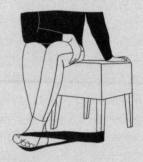

and resisting the pull of the band. Perform with control, through full range. Swap sides between sets. This exercise can be quite uncomfortable on a bare foot, so I recommend wearing shoes. But if you do so, make sure the band wraps around the big toe area of the shoe and not the middle.

PERFORM 2–3 X 12–15 REPS PER LEG.

# PERFORMANCE PLAN

You'll need access to weights for the exercises in this workout – barbells, dumbbells or kettlebells are ideal. Your own bodyweight won't provide sufficient overload to promote strength (and if it does feel challenging without weights then you should turn to the Foundation Plan on p. 164.) Some exercises can be performed using gym equipment (such as the Smith machine and leg press) instead of free weights.

The weight or resistance used should be challenging, but don't overdo it – it needn't be so heavy that you 'fail' (reach fatigue and cannot continue) by the last repetition but the last couple of reps should be difficult. Perform the exercises with control and focus. When you can reach the higher end of the recommended reps and sets range, increase the weight or follow any progressions suggested. Research suggests strength training two to three times per week for 10 weeks to gain benefits. After that, you can maintain what you've got with just one session per week. Make sure you don't do more than one session per week during the Specific phase of your marathon-training plan.

Try to keep these workouts separate from hard or long runs. Aim to allow a minimum of nine hours between the two modalities.

## Squat with barbell
*glute and quad strength, ankle flexibility*

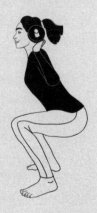

Stand with your feet a little wider than hip-distance apart, toes forwards or turning slightly outwards. Position a barbell across your upper back, your handgrip slightly wider than shoulder width. Send your hips back and descend into a squat, keeping the knees in line with the toes ('pressing' the knees outwards can help), until your thighs are roughly parallel to the ground or until you can no longer maintain a neutral spine position (i.e. you see/feel yourself rounding or arching your back). Stand up quickly by driving through the heels and glutes to return to a standing position.
PERFORM 3 X 5–8 REPS WITH 2 MINS' RECOVERY BETWEEN SETS.

## Deadlift with barbell

*strengthens hamstrings and glutes, challenges hip extension while keeping knee joint stable*

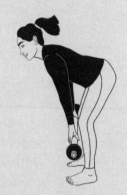

Stand with your feet below your hips, holding a barbell with your handgrip slightly wider than shoulder width, palms facing your thighs. Bend your knees just a little and make sure your bodyweight is mostly under the balls of your feet, not your heels. Now 'hinge' at the hips, by pushing your bottom back, keeping your spine in a neutral position. Keep the bar close to your legs as you lower it to your shins, then return to standing by pressing your hips forwards. Don't bend and straighten your knees – they should stay slightly bent throughout. Allow your head to stay in line with your spine rather than facing forwards throughout the movement.

PERFORM 3 X 5–8 REPS WITH 2 MINS' RECOVERY BETWEEN SETS.

## Hip thrust with barbell

*focused glute work, challenges control of pelvic position*

Support your upper back on a bench or chair with your feet hip-width apart, your knees bent to 90 degrees (your body should be in a straight line from your knees to your shoulders). Hold a barbell or weight plate securely across your hips. Leading with the hips, lower your bottom towards the ground, then press up through your heels to extend the hips back to a straight line between your knees, hips and shoulders. If your hamstrings cramp up, slightly straighten the knee; this is a hint that you are not using your bottom muscles enough! To progress, you can perform the exercise on a single leg, with the other knee lifted.

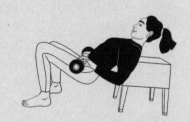

PERFORM 3 X 5–8 REPS WITH 2 MINS' RECOVERY BETWEEN SETS.

## Split squat

*eccentric quad strength, challenges balance and hip-knee-ankle alignment*

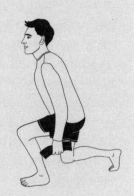

With a barbell across your upper back (held with hands slightly wider than shoulder width apart) or dumbbells in each hand, take a large step forwards, so that your front foot is flat but the rear heel is lifted. Keep your torso above your hips. Lower your hips towards the floor by bending at both knees, until the front thigh is roughly parallel with the ground and the rear knee hovers above the ground. Don't bend your front knee deeper than 90 degrees. Push down through the heel of the front foot to return to the standing position.

You can progress this exercise by elevating the rear foot on a low bench or chair.

PERFORM 2–3 X 5–8 REPS PER LEG WITH 2 MINS' RECOVERY BETWEEN SETS.

## Standing calf raises

*calf and ankle strength, stability and mobility*

The best way to 'weight' a calf raise is with a heavy backpack. I've got one full of exercise physiology textbooks specifically for the job! Otherwise, you can hold a dumbbell in the hand on the side you are working.

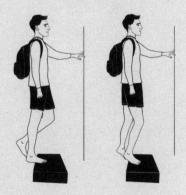

Stand tall with just the front half of your right foot on a step, the other leg dangling freely. Drop the right heel down below the level of the step, bending the knee at the same time. Now lift the heel above the level of the step (so you're on tiptoe), only straightening the knee at the top of the movement. Return to the start position for the next rep. Switch legs between sets.

If you have heel or Achilles issues, perform this movement from a flat surface instead of a step. (i.e. bend the knee, extend through the ankle, then straighten the knee at the top of the movement.)

PERFORM 2–3 X 8–12 REPS PER LEG WITH 2 MINS' RECOVERY BETWEEN SETS.

## Step-up
*improved landing control, balance*

Stand in front of a step or sturdy surface (approximately 30cm/12in tall) that you can step up on to safely. Place the left foot flat on the step (a). Hold a barbell across your upper back or a dumbbell in each hand. Now drive through your left foot to straighten the leg (b). Let your right leg simply hang. Initiate the descent by pushing your hips backwards, rather than your knee forwards. Control the descent until your right foot lands lightly. Repeat. Swap sides between sets.

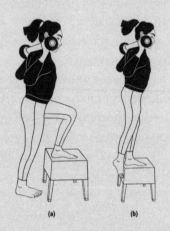

(a)          (b)

You can progress this exercise by increasing the weight or raising the height of the step (don't go beyond the height at which you have a 90-degree bend at the knee).

PERFORM 2–3 X 5–8 REPS PER LEG WITH 2 MINS' RECOVERY BETWEEN SETS.

# Leaping to the next level

Plyometric or 'reactive' strength training is about harnessing 'free' energy, by optimising the use of the elasticity of tendons and other connective tissue. Using this free energy means that muscles don't have to produce as much force, making movement less costly in terms of energy. One study found that plyometric training helped to improve running economy by 4.1 per cent over nine weeks, while a running-only group showed no improvement.

Plyometric movements entail an eccentric (lengthening) contraction followed immediately by a (concentric) shortening one, known as the stretch-shortening cycle. The former stores energy; the latter releases it, just like when an archer draws back their bow to fire an arrow.

The running stride itself is plyometric: if you think what happens when your foot strikes the ground, the muscles around the ankle and knee (the calves and quads) have to lengthen to control (resist) your body's downward movement and prevent you collapsing to the floor, before shortening again to propel you forwards.

In between these two phases, there is a split-second moment when the muscle is neither lengthening nor shortening (this is called the 'amortisation' phase) and this is when the potential energy is highest. The more rapidly you can 'switch' from the eccentric to the concentric contraction, the more you can make use of the stored energy. I keep talking about muscular contractions, but it's actually the tendons – the cords of connective tissue that attach muscles to bones – that store the energy.

When a tendon is lengthened, its relatively stiff structure and low tolerance to stretching make it want to return to its resting length as soon as possible. The body capitalises on this this by using the tendons (especially the Achilles tendon) to store and release energy, hence reducing the amount of muscular work that needs to be done to propel the body forwards.

The plyometric exercises below help improve the tendons' capacity to store and release energy as well as improving neural input (the nervous system's sensitivity and responsiveness). Perform these once or twice per week during the Development Phase of the marathon-training plans, but only once you've done at least 10–12 weeks of regular strength and conditioning. They can be done as part of a set of running drills, or after a warm-up, before you run.

In all three exercises, pull your toes back towards your shins (dorsiflex the foot) to create some pre-tension in your calf muscles. Aim to be 'stiff' in your ankles and knees before you land.

### 1. Pogo jump

Standing tall, with your feet below your hips, perform six vertical jumps in quick succession. Aim to jump as high as you can and spend as little time on the ground as possible between jumps, keeping your ankles and knees relatively stiff on landing.

PERFORM 2–3 SETS X 6 JUMPS WITH 2 MINS' RECOVERY BETWEEN SETS.

### 2. Drop jump

Stand on a box 20–30cm (8–12in) high. Hold one leg a little way in front of you, allowing your bodyweight to shift forwards until you have to step off. Land with both feet and as soon as you strike the ground, rebound vertically. Again, the aim is to spend as little time on the ground and to jump as high as possible. Repeat. (Make sure you step off, rather than jumping off.)

PERFORM 2–3 SETS X 6 JUMPS (STEP OFF WITH THE OTHER FOOT ON THE SECOND SET WITH 2 MINS' RECOVERY BETWEEN SETS).

### 3. Hop and stick

Stand tall and lift one foot away from the ground. Bend your supporting leg into a quarter squat, and then perform an explosive hop forwards, aiming to travel as far as possible (not upwards) and to 'stick' the landing without losing your balance. There should only be a small bend at the knee, ankle and hip on landing. Now turn around and hop back, on the same foot. Perform six single hops in total before switching legs.

As this gets easier, you can join two hops together, then three, all the way up to the point where you string all six together.

PERFORM 2–3 SETS X 6 HOPS PER LEG WITH 2 MINS' RECOVERY BETWEEN SETS.

# 12
# STAYING HEALTHY

## Avoiding those occupational hazards

There is a bell-shaped curve relationship between running and immune system function. A moderate amount of exercise is associated with optimal immune functioning, but if you don't exercise at all – or if you exercise too much – your immune system can be rendered less effective. During marathon training, most of us are pushing the boundaries of our usual training load and are therefore more likely to be putting our immune systems under stress. That makes us more susceptible to colds and other infections, just when we need to be on top form. So, what can you do to avoid getting sick?

### Can I train with a cold?

There's nothing wrong with training with a mild cold. If you're not sure, a brief, easy run is the best way to find out if you feel up to it. 'Above the neck' symptoms, such as a stuffy head, runny nose or mild sore throat should be fine. But 'below the neck' symptoms such as aches and pains or a cough should be seen as red flags. Get some rest. And never train if you have a temperature. Training through illness can not only delay your recovery and prolong the time you have off running, it can also be dangerous, leading to inflammation of the heart muscle (myocarditis).

Sufficient rest and sleep play a huge role in maintaining healthy immunity (see Chapter 9 for a reminder). A healthy diet does, too, with a particular emphasis on what you eat in the two hours following any very hard or very long run, when your immune system will be most severely suppressed. Consuming carbohydrate (30–60g/1–2oz per hour) *during* these training sessions also helps mitigate the hit the immune system takes. Read more about marathon nutrition in Chapter 17.

Be extra vigilant about hygiene during marathon training: wash your hands regularly and thoroughly or use hand sanitiser if you don't have access to water, avoid touching public surfaces like stair rails and door handles where possible, and minimise your exposure to crowds (especially of children!). If the latter is unavoidable, consider using a nasal spray like First Defence when you're in company. A study of Norwegian athletes found that air travel presented a particularly high risk in terms of suppressing the immune system. The elevated risk lasted a full week after flying. You may not be able to avoid this, but it is worth knowing, just in case you can factor it into any travel plans.

## Running ills

There are some common conditions and afflictions that running makes us more vulnerable to – especially the long runs of marathon training. While none of them is life-threatening, they can make training more arduous and uncomfortable, so it's useful to know how to address them – or even better, avoid them. Here's an alphabetical guide. . .

### Athlete's foot

Athlete's foot is a fungal infection that loves warm, damp places. It is more likely to take hold on cracked or damaged skin, so it isn't any wonder it attacks runners' feet. To avoid this painful and itchy condition, never linger in sweaty footwear post-run. Wash and thoroughly dry your feet (including between the toes) and let them get some air by going barefoot (unless you already have symptoms) or wearing open footwear. At the first sign of trouble, try dabbing tea tree oil, an antifungal, between your toes or use an antifungal spray, cream or powder. Remember that your shoe insoles may also harbour the infection: soak them in a tea tree oil solution or spray them with an antifungal spray – or replace them.

If you are a regular sufferer, bamboo and merino wool socks have natural antibacterial properties – and some synthetic socks have copper or silver threads woven into them, which are antibacterial and antifungal. Always wear flip-flops in public areas (especially damp places like gym changing rooms and pool edges) as athlete's foot is highly contagious.

## Blisters

Blisters are a build-up of fluid between the upper and lower layers of the skin, caused by friction between your skin and your shoes or socks. You may find that even if you've never suffered with blisters before, long runs bring them on. This could be due to more prolonged rubbing, more moisture and heat around your feet or changes to your running form as you get tired.

If you are troubled by blisters, pay particular attention to shoe fit and the type of socks you choose (seamless socks with sweat-wicking properties are best – some runners swear by double-layer socks or toe socks for blister prevention).

If specific areas always suffer, take preventative action by covering them with zinc oxide tape or moleskin *before* running, to protect them. Some people like to use a lubricant, such as Vaseline or Bodyglide, to prevent blister-causing friction – but don't apply so much that your toes are slipping around in your socks. If you get a blister, leave it for 24 hours to see if the fluid is reabsorbed. If not, you could opt to pop it, using a sterilised needle. Pierce the blister close to the edge, to safeguard the skin covering it. Drain the fluid and dab the blister with antiseptic, then cover it with a blister plaster or gauze pad to protect it from bacteria while it heals. NB: only cover it when you're in shoes – otherwise, allow the air to get to it to help dry it out.

## Black toenails

If you find your big toenails turning black during marathon training, you certainly won't be alone. As many as a quarter of distance runners suffer from this and it is often regarded as a badge of honour. The blackness comes from bruising beneath the nail as a result of the repeated forward movement of the toe inside the shoe. Shoes that are too small can cause this, but so can shoes that allow the foot to slide forwards too much, or running downhill, when there is more forward motion of the foot inside the shoe. Sometimes, the cause is unrelated to shoe fit and is simply a result of increased mileage creating increased repetitive trauma. Building up your mileage gradually can help prevent this.

The best way to deal with a black toenail is to do nothing. It will either fall off when it's ready or grow out. But if it's causing you significant pain, it's worth seeing a podiatrist or your GP to relieve the pressure behind the nail by lancing it. Don't be tempted to do this yourself.

## Chafing

A recent study found that 14 per cent of runners had suffered chafing within the last year. Chafing is caused by something rubbing against the skin for a prolonged period – clothing, equipment or other body parts. It's more likely to happen when you and your clothing are wet, either as a result of sweating or rainfall.

The right defence depends on the afflicted area. Nipples are best protected by proprietary nipple guards or surgical tape, but if it's a larger area, such as your armpits or inner thighs that rub, use an anti-chafing lubricant or consider clothing coverage (a sleeved, seamless, tight-fitting base layer; compression-type shorts or running tights).

Lubricants come in a range of forms, from balm and gel to powder and spray (see Resources). Good-fitting garments and gear are less likely to chafe, so think about issues such as arm-hole size, waistband style, seam placement, fabric type and the potential for adjustability when you're buying new kit.

If you do get rubbed up the wrong way, gently wash the affected area and apply a healing cream, such as Sudocrem.

## Muscle cramp

You probably don't need me to tell you that cramp is a painful and involuntary muscle contraction. One study found that 18 per cent of runners experienced cramp during a marathon.

There is still much debate about why it happens, with sport scientists falling into two camps. In the blue corner, there are those who believe the most probable cause is fatigue or 'overload' of the neuromuscular system, which creates an imbalance between excitatory (activating) and inhibitory (deactivating) signals from the central nervous system to the offending muscle. This can occur during exercise in the absence of substantial sweat loss or disturbance of electrolyte balance. In the red corner, scientists point to studies showing that cramp is more prevalent when a bodyweight loss of 3 per cent occurs compared to no, or lesser, bodyweight losses. They also cite studies that suggest that during prolonged exertion in a hot environment (where both sweat loss and water intake are high), increased sodium intake can significantly reduce the incidence of cramp. In a classic 1936 study, 12,000 men working in a steel mill, where cramp was widespread, were given a saline solution to drink, while men at a neighbouring mill continued to receive plain water. The saline almost eliminated the problem, while cramp was not abated among those given water – with many cases so bad they required hospitalisation. In 2021, a study at Edith Cowan University in Australia found that an oral rehydration solution (containing electrolytes) decreased muscle cramp susceptibility in runners, while water did not.

If the neuromuscular fatigue theory is correct, the incidence of cramp should decline as you get fitter and more comfortable with long runs; and while some studies have found this to be true, it doesn't always seem to be the case. Be mindful about how quickly you build up your running speed and distance, to give time for your nervous and muscular systems to adapt. I would also recommend experimenting with electrolytes if you have a serious problem with cramp. Anecdotally, I know regular cramp sufferers who have alleviated the problem significantly by using electrolytes, or even salt tablets. Maybe in the future, researchers will find a link between neuromuscular fatigue and electrolyte levels in some runners (such as those who are salty sweaters, *see* p. 241).

If cramp does strike while you're running, the best solution is to stretch; cramp most often strikes muscles that cross two joints, such as the calves (which cross the ankle and the knee), so make sure you address both the relevant joints in your remedial stretch.

## Side stitches

Everyone gets a side stitch now and again – a 2015 study reported that in a single running event, one in five participants could be expected to suffer a stitch (known as exercise-related transient abdominal pain or ETAP).

Although scientists don't believe that a side stitch is entirely down to the jolting nature of running, the incidence is 10 times higher among runners than in cyclists. Unfortunately, no single cause – or solution – has yet been identified; but there are a number of factors worth exploring.

First, keep your core muscles strong. A weak core puts more stress on the diaphragm, the muscle that facilitates breathing, which can cause it to fatigue or go into spasm.

Consider your posture. A study in the *Journal of Science and Medicine* found that a stiff thoracic spine (upper back) and kyphotic posture (where the upper spine curves forwards) were both associated with a higher incidence of stitches, leading the researchers to recommend postural exercises to address these shortfalls. Rolling out your upper back on a foam roller before a run, and stretching out over it (with the roller positioned lengthways down your back) afterwards will help mobilise your thoracic spine.

Also think about what and when you eat before a run. Irritation of the peritoneum, a double-layered, fluid-filled sheath surrounding the abdominal cavity, has been implicated in causing stitches. It's thought that a bloated stomach – resulting from eating too close to running, or taking on too much fluid at once – can push against the inner layer of the peritoneum.

Another possible mechanism behind a stitch, also related to the peritoneum, is a reduction in the amount of fluid separating the two layers. This could be due to dehydration.

To minimise the risks, avoid running within two hours of a meal and stick to small portion sizes. Make sure you stay hydrated, but using a 'little and often' drinking strategy. Also consider *what* you drink. Research in the *International Journal of Sports Nutrition and Exercise Metabolism* found that fruit juice caused more bloating and stitches than did a proprietary isotonic sports drink.

What about remedial action? Well, there's nothing very scientific on offer. Some runners find it helpful to switch their breathing pattern to exhale as the foot on the opposite side to the stitch lands (for example, if your stitch is on the right, you exhale as your left foot hits the ground). Others find that breathing deeply, or reaching the arms overhead and stretching sideways – away from the side stitch – helps. I recommend slowing your pace as much as you need to until the stitch passes. I also find it helpful to gently knead the sore area. See if any of these options work for you.

# Tummy trouble (aka 'runner's trots')

No athlete is immune to gastrointestinal (GI) disturbances (which include gut discomfort, cramping, flatulence, a sudden and urgent need to 'go' and diarrhoea) but the fact that runners suffer more widely than cyclists suggests that the up-and-down motion does play a role. A recent survey found that 62 per cent of runners have had to stop mid run for a poo. Twelve per cent said they'd got caught short, experiencing faecal incontinence during a run.

Other likely factors behind gastrointestinal discomfort include the diversion of blood flow from the guts to the working muscles, sensitivity to specific food or beverage types, and dehydration (a recent study found that problems were more prevalent even when runners were only 'hypo-hydrated', i.e. mildly dehydrated). The incidence and severity of symptoms is significantly higher when exercising in hot conditions, and while you can't change the weather, you might find that tweaking your pre- and in-run fuelling strategy (for example, changing what and how much you drink) helps. One small study found that four weeks of probiotic supplementation slightly reduced gastrointestinal symptoms in runners training in the heat and also mitigated the effects of the heat on their performance.

So what else can you do to stop GI distress? If you aren't managing to empty your bowels before you run, this is the first line of defence. Try to establish a poo-triggering routine before training runs and races, so that your bowels can perform on cue. This might include eating something, drinking a coffee and some light activity.

For those who are plagued by the trots even after having visited the toilet pre-run, the secret is figuring out what it is that's irritating your guts. Keep a 'food and toilet' diary alongside your training journal for a while, to see if you can find a pattern. Some common gut irritants include caffeine, alcohol, fibre, sugar, artificial sweeteners and dairy products. Non-steroidal anti-inflammatories (NSAIDS) – especially on an empty stomach – can also sensitise the stomach.

Here are a few other tips for those who suffer from GI symptoms:

☑ Allow longer between eating and running than you are currently. And if you run in the mornings, try allowing longer between getting up and beginning the run.

- ☑ Experiment with different energy products – for example, swap gels for sports drinks, or real food for gels.
- ☑ Try drinking a little more fluid, either before or during your run.
- ☑ Try training at a different time of day (though bear in mind you'll likely be racing in the morning).
- ☑ If you experience GI pain during a run, slow down to a walk – the symptoms and that urge to 'go' may just pass.
- ☑ If you are really concerned about race day, you could consider using an anti-diarrhoea formulation. If you plan to do this, try it on a long training run first to check if it works and doesn't cause any unwanted side effects. Don't make this a regular practice, however – it's much better to get to the cause than prevent the symptoms.

# 13

# RUNNING AWAY FROM INJURY

## Injury prevention and action

There's an old runners' joke that says we have only three states of being: injured, recovering from injury or about to get injured. It's true that running does have a high incidence of injury, although the word is used to cover a broad spectrum of afflictions, from a niggly hip to a sprained ankle. The latter is classed as an 'acute' injury, because it occurs suddenly with a clear cause. But the vast majority of injuries befalling runners come under the 'chronic' category; they creep up on you over time (perhaps over the length of a run, or over a few days or even weeks) without an obvious cause. While they may seemingly have come out of nowhere, there are usually signs to heed (*see* 'Listen to your body' on p. 186) and some element of either overuse or misuse at the root.

So what can you do to avoid becoming one of the high percentage of runners who get injured each year? Well, while you can't completely eliminate the risk (just look how often elite runners succumb to injury) there are many steps you can take to reduce your risk and to prevent troublesome niggles from becoming anything more serious.

# Train right

In my experience, when runners get injured, they often blame 'not stretching enough' or wearing the 'wrong' shoes. But by far the biggest contributing factor to running injuries is training error. These errors usually boil down to increasing volume and/or intensity too quickly, doing too much overall (relative to your current fitness level) or not allowing enough rest and recovery time. That's why abiding by those training principles is so important and why your training plan should be built around them – and you.

If you miss some of your marathon training – whether through illness, or just taking your eye off the ball temporarily – don't try to 'make up time' by cramming in the sessions you skipped. And if you've lost a few weeks, don't jump ahead to where you should now be on the programme – go back to where you were and build from there. Yes, you may end up behind where you wanted to be, but that's safer than ending up injured and not being able to run at all.

Rest and recovery – be it immediately after a session or more broadly within your training programme – is all part of training right, too. *See* Chapter 9 for more details on what helps and hinders the recovery process.

# Run right

We looked at the benefits of improving running form in Chapter 10. As well as conserving energy, good form lowers the risk of overloading, and thereby irritating, specific areas of the body: for example, increasing cadence reduces load on the knees. Maintaining adequate strength and flexibility also helps your body cope with the forces of running and hold on to good technique as you get tired. A 2017 study found that strengthening the hip muscles reduced the risk of IT band problems.

What about footwear? The jury is still out on whether shoe choice influences injury risk – research suggests that while most runners believe it to be an important factor, health care professionals rate it less so – and it's easy to see why, when you look at the conflicting findings. One recent study found no difference in injury risk between using a shoe with a high heel-toe drop or a low heel-toe. Another (co-funded by a sportswear brand) found that runners with 'pronated' feet experienced fewer injuries when wearing a motion control shoe – in direct contrast to an earlier study that found no association between a pronated foot type and injury rate over the course of a year.

There's more about footwear in Chapter 7, but there are two important points to be made here: first, if you develop an injury and have recently changed your shoe type or model, it's certainly worth considering this as a possible cause (and mentioning it to any sports medicine professional you go to see). Second, having more than one pair of shoes 'on the go' appears to help keep injuries at bay. A study published in the *Scandinavian Journal of Medicine and Science in Sports* found that rotating two or more pairs of shoes was associated with fewer injuries among runners. (A great fact to tell your other half if they complain about how much you spend on running kit!) The reason why changing your footwear from run to run might be protective is that it subtly changes the load on the musculoskeletal system. Running on a variety of different surfaces – mixing road with trail, hilly with flat – is a sensible measure for the exact same reason. Read more about running surfaces and terrain on p. 93.

## Eat right

A well-nourished body can withstand the rigours of training better than an undernourished one. A healthy diet that provides enough energy (calories) and nutrients is vitally important, both in terms of avoiding injuries and in making a successful recovery from them.

In the elite echelons of the sport, marathon runners tend to be slim and slight. But this is largely down to natural selection and it doesn't mean all of us should be striving to be as light as possible. Research links inadequate calorie intake to a raised risk of injury, with a particularly strong association to stress fractures. In women athletes, the factor most associated with injury risk is fat intake, revealing a misconception that unlike carbohydrate and protein, fat is an undesirable nutrient for a runner. If you find yourself losing weight during marathon training, keep an eye on it and be aware that more weight loss isn't necessarily better.

There's lots more information on nutrition for marathon training, racing and recovery in Section 6.

# Listen to your body

Before we leave the topic of injury avoidance behind, I hope it's not too annoying to say that one of the best solutions is to nip problems in the bud. So often, we ignore minor niggles until they become unignorable. As running coach Malcolm Balk says: 'listen to the whispers and you won't have to hear the screams.'

Knowing how to distinguish 'good' pain from 'bad' pain is an important part of listening to your body. Post-run generalised soreness and aches are characteristic of good pain, which indicates that you worked hard, successfully overloaded your body and now need to recover. Bad pain, on the other hand, is a sign that you did something too hard, for too long, or that you did it badly. This kind of pain is likely to be located in one specific area, causing you to change the way you walk or run and instead of easing off over time, it lingers or gets worse.

# I'm injured! What now?

Let's imagine that despite your best efforts to avoid injury, you've got a niggle, or worse. What should you do?

The 'first port of call' answer to this question used to be so simple – spelled out in the acronym RICE: rest, ice, compress, elevate. But several sports medicine experts – including Dr Gabe Mirkin, the sports medicine doctor who coined RICE back in 1978 – now believe that RICE is not the best approach to injuries. 'It appears that both complete rest and ice may delay healing, instead of helping,' Mirkin writes on his website. 'Don't increase your pain, but you want to move as soon as you can.'

While a couple of days of no running or less running can be useful if you've just overdone things and ended up sore, the idea that rest 'cures' injuries is misplaced. If you think back to the SAID principle – the concept that the body adapts to the demands we place on it – taking a week off gives the body a signal that it no longer needs to be able to deal with the demands of running. This results in deconditioning, leaving the niggling part *less* likely to be able to cope with running once you return to it, rather than *more* likely.

Let's be clear: I am not saying that you should ignore injuries or run through intense pain. But rather than resting (as in doing no activity), you need to find a way to 'load' the injured area to an appropriate extent and in a controlled, progressive manner. This loading is essential for healthy muscles, tendons and bones and is part of the healing process.

Appropriate loading might mean a reduced volume and/or intensity of running, replacing running with cross-training, or concentrating on specific rehabilitation exercises. Or a combination of all three. Ideally, this is best figured out with the help of a sports medicine professional, although in my experience, many are too quick to prescribe 'rest'.

In a study published in the *American Journal of Sports Medicine*, athletes with Achilles tendinopathy were divided into two groups. One group followed a strength-based rehab programme for the Achilles and calf muscles, while the other group followed the rehab programme *and* continued their sport, even if it involved tendon-loading activities like running. The rules were that their pain should not exceed a score of 5 out of 10 (*see* 'Stop on red' on the following page) and should have settled by the next morning. After six weeks, improvement in function and reduction in pain level were the same in both groups. Similar research in 2017 looked at runners with knee pain. They were either prescribed strength exercises or gait retraining to help improve their condition. Some were advised on how to modify their running to keep it within acceptable pain levels during the rehab, while others did no running. Both groups gained the same amount of symptom relief and functional improvement over an eight-week period.

A pain rating scale, like the one on the following page, will enable you to make a sensible decision about whether – and how much – you can continue running while you address an injury. A minor niggle may settle with a reduced volume or intensity that gradually builds back up, and never rear its ugly head again – other issues may require a break from running and a more managed rehabilitation.

## Getting help

When you consult a physiotherapist, or other sports practitioner, go armed with information. How long has your niggle been niggling? Does it hurt every time you run, or just when you run fast, or up hills? Maybe it only hurts after you've finished. Or it hurts pretty much all the time. Did anything coincide with its onset – such as an increase in volume or intensity? A different pair of shoes or running surface? What have you tried so far to ease it? That's your side of the bargain.

## STOP ON RED

This numerical pain rating scale (NPRS) will help you decide whether to run or rest. Think of it as a traffic light system:

　　0–2 Safe zone (green)
　　2–5 Acceptable zone (amber)
　　6–10 Excessive zone (red)

- The pain can score up to '5' on the NPRS during the activity. But be wary of escalating pain. If your pain starts off at a '1' but creeps up to 5 or beyond, you need to back off.
- You should be running in your usual way. Running in a different or awkward way to try to avoid irritating the niggle may eventually cause problems elsewhere.
- A pain rating of 5 is acceptable on completion of the activity provided it settles within 24 hours.
- Pain and stiffness should not be increasing from week to week.

Now on to theirs. Ensure that you leave the clinic with a clear idea of what your problem is, what the likely cause is and what action you need to take, both to hasten recovery and to prevent it happening again. Expect to get some 'homework' (I always steer clear of therapists who simply stick some sort of machine on you, rather than properly engaging with you and the issue you are presenting), and ensure you know exactly how to do any strengthening or mobilising exercises you are given, and how often to do them. Don't be afraid to take notes or ask for diagrams, if it helps. Alternatively, get them to film themselves/you doing the exercise on your phone so you go away with a visual reference.

Discuss whether you can maintain running at some level while your niggly area settles down. If they recommend no running, ask for an idea of how long you will be out for and how many appointments they anticipate you will need. Be wary if your treatment seems to be going on and on, without any signs of the injury improving – discuss this with them or go elsewhere. And finally, do what you're told! There is no sense in paying good money for expert advice if you don't heed it.

## Be patient

The dos and don'ts outlined on the following pages will help you make the best progress with settling an injury. But the biggest healer of all is time – the one thing that a runner in marathon training doesn't have much of. Depending on the nature of the injury, and how much running and/or cross-training you are able to do during your rehabilitation period, you may need to review your marathon goal once you are back in training. Or you may decide to defer or delay your race. What's really important is that you only return to training when you are ready. There's nothing more frustrating than starting back, only to find that you're back on the bench two to three weeks later. I found physiotherapist Tom Goom's advice on returning to running really helpful and share it here.

# READY TO RUN CHECKLIST

If you have had some time off running through injury, physiotherapist Tom Goom recommends you can tick all the boxes below before you try a run...

☑ There is minimal pain or no pain during day-to-day activities.

☑ A 30-minute walk feels fine.

☑ You can jog on the spot for one minute without pain.

If you can tick all the boxes, you're in a good position to go for a run and see how it feels. 'There is always some trial and error involved in trying to find the appropriate amount of running to do,' says Tom. 'It's best to start low – with something that feels really manageable – and build up. You're aiming to find a distance and pace where pain is minimal during the run (e.g. 0–3 out of 10) and settles quickly afterwards (back to normal within 24 hours). If your symptoms kick in during the run, note where you are time- or distance-wise and call it a day. Then wait to see how it responds the next day. If the pain settles, you can run again, but this time, stop a little before the time/distance you were at when symptoms occurred previously. For example, if pain started at 3½ miles (5.6km), run 3 miles (4.8km) next time and gradually build from there.'

# 10 Dos and don'ts for injured runners

⊗ Don't stretch injured muscles. This will only cause more damage to the injured tissues. You can gently move the joint through its range, if pain allows, but don't hold stretches.

☑ Do ice for pain relief, if you like, but only in short bouts and not to enable you to mask pain so you can run. A 2017 study found that icing for 10 minutes was just as effective as longer periods in reducing swelling and pain. Lengthy applications are more likely to interfere with the natural inflammatory response that is part of the healing process.

⊗ Don't take painkillers to enable you to run. If you do take painkillers, avoid anti-inflammatories (especially over the first 48 hours) such as ibuprofen, which has been shown to reduce muscle protein synthesis and delay healing. A recent study suggests most runners do precisely the opposite, with more than 70 per cent using NSAIDS for injuries. Paracetamol is a better choice.

☑ Do make sure you are consuming enough protein. Injured runners require 1.5–2g protein/kg of bodyweight (1.5–2g/2.2lb) per day, spread throughout the day in meals and snacks rather than in just one or two hits. This extra protein is needed to stimulate muscle protein synthesis and to decrease the loss in muscle mass associated with less or no training.

⊗ Don't be tempted to cut your calorie intake too drastically for fear of gaining weight. A study in the journal *Nutrition in Clinical Practice* shows that the healing process itself requires a lot of energy.

☑ Do approach your rehab with the same attitude as you would your training. Every rehab session counts, and you should give it your full attention and effort. Note down how you do each time, so you can gauge whether you are progressing.

⊗ Don't rely on someone else to 'fix' you. Manual therapy, such as massage or physio, can be very helpful, but in almost every case, you'll need to do some work yourself – be it strength work, running drills, mobility or stability.

☑ Do consider getting your vitamin D status checked. Research suggests that low vitamin D is associated with an increased risk of stress fractures. *See* p. 250 for more information. Other research links low calcium levels with stress fractures and low bone density. However, there's likely not much to be gained from supplementation if you are not deficient in these particular nutrients.

☒ Don't rush into having scans, such as ultrasound or MRI. Pain and damage are not the same thing. To illustrate the point, MRI scans of the knees of 44 people suffering no pain revealed meniscal (cartilage) degeneration or tears in almost every case. Other research found that 38 per cent of pain-free subjects showed abnormalities (such as 'bulging' discs) in the lumbar spine. These are the kinds of scan results that are used to 'explain' pain – but the subjects in these studies were not suffering any pain, demonstrating the potential problems associated with relying on a scan to tell you why you're hurting.

☑ Do consider taping. You can't have failed to notice the number of elite athletes who compete covered in strips of brightly coloured kinesio tape these days. The efficacy of taping isn't clear-cut in the scientific research. While one study on knee osteoarthritis found that it provided no benefit in either pain reduction or joint function, another found that it did reduce pain levels in runners suffering from patellofemoral pain. Equally, one study found that taping could improve proprioception after ankle sprains, while another concluded its use was not warranted in treating shin splints. So why am I suggesting it? It's relatively cheap and you can apply it yourself, for one thing. But also, studies using 'sham' application of tape as a comparison to 'correct' application have found that both can be effective in reducing perception of pain, allowing rehabilitation exercises to be performed more comfortably. So, there's an argument that simply putting on some tape can help, even if it's just a psychological sticking plaster...

# ON YOUR MARKS

# 14

# CHOOSING THE RIGHT RACE

## What to consider when picking your event

For most runners, the marathon conjures up images of big-city events like London, Berlin, New York and Boston. These iconic races are pretty special, but they are notoriously difficult to get into – and far from the only options on the table.

Race search website Let's Do This lists dozens of marathons in the UK alone – there are alternative big-city races to consider in every part of the country, from Brighton to Belfast; large road-based events in more remote locations, like Snowdonia and Loch Ness; and small-town – but highly regarded – races in Abingdon and Halstead. There's also a growing number of off-road events, like Beachy Head, that take you up hill and down dale. Expand your search overseas and the choice becomes overwhelming.

I know it can be disheartening if you've set your sights on London, or one of the Marathon Majors, and haven't been able to secure a place, but there can be advantages in taking part in a lesser-known event. A smaller race is likely to involve less hassle at every stage – from getting a place and registering to finding accommodation to getting to the start and queuing for the loo! You may even have a better chance of achieving your goal time, thanks to less congestion on the course. On the other hand, less well-established races may be less slickly organised – and smaller races tend to have fewer spectators, which some runners can find disheartening.

## Do your research

That's why it pays to do your research. There are many factors to consider when choosing the right race – it's not all about the medal – from time of year to location, the size (and ability) of the field and the route itself. Do as much groundwork as you can, looking at race websites, asking other runners and poring over race reviews – if you're in doubt about something, contact the race organisers to ask (it'll give you an insight into how well organised they are).

When thinking about what time of year the race is, you need to consider the likely weather conditions both in terms of the training and race day. Most marathons are held in spring and autumn, to increase the chances of good running conditions (southern Europe is a great option for late-season races right through to November) but there are some events in which wintry weather and tough conditions are considered all part of the challenge.

Also consider how long the race date leaves you for training – is it long enough to get adequately prepared and do the race justice?

## QUESTIONS TO ASK BEFORE YOU SIGN UP...

- Do you have to register in person? If so, is it before race day? (You need to factor this in to your travel plans.)
- How many drinks stations are there? What do they offer?
- What time of day is the race held? (This may have a bearing on the time you need to get up as well as the weather conditions.)
- Will it be easy for your supporters to make their way to different points along the course?
- What are the logistics like for getting to the start and, more importantly, from the finish?
- Is there a race cut-off time and if so, are you comfortable with it?
- What is the policy for withdrawal or deferral?

## Location, location, location

Think carefully about location when you are selecting a race. Running Boston might sound amazing but have you factored in how you might deal with travel fatigue or jet lag? (You may need to build in more time to your travel plans.) Do you have willing friends or family to accompany you and if not, are you sure you're OK without anyone cheering you on? In my experience, it's definitely worth considering booking a race package if you are taking part in an overseas race. This will typically include your race entry fee, along with accommodation and travel. Not having to think about how to get to registration, where to eat and how to travel to the start takes away much of the pre-race stress and helps you conserve energy for the race you've travelled all that way for.

Even if you're running a UK race, location is relevant. A long journey will either entail overnight accommodation (adding to the budget) or a very early start on race day, which can have consequences on your performance. It all needs to be considered.

## Who's in?

One of the pluses of mega events like London and New York is that you can be pretty sure that runners of every type will be represented – from serious podium contenders to club runners, fancy-dress-clad charity runners to slow-but-sure plodders. This vast spread is less likely to be found at smaller events (and is less common in Europe, where more runners tend to be 'serious' ones). Depending on your point of view, this could be a benefit or a drawback. So, as well as thinking about the number of runners in the race you're contemplating, consider the 'quality' of the field, too. A look at previous years' results is helpful, as well as checking whether the race has a set cut-off time.

## Right on course

Finally, consider the route itself. If you are chasing a PB, you'll be looking for flat races without too many twists and turns, little exposure to wind, and wide, uncrowded roads. Many of the big-city marathons – including London, Berlin and Chicago – are pancake flat, others use the word 'flat' in their race descriptions in what I'd call a more creative manner!

Other route issues to consider are the quality of the surface underfoot (London's tarmac is said to be easier on the joints than New York's concrete while Rome is infamous for its cobblestones), the altitude (Madrid boasts Europe's highest city marathon) and the view. More than 45 per cent of people in a survey said that the scenery was an important consideration when choosing a race, so it's worth a second thought. While Rotterdam is renowned as one of the fastest marathons in the world, it's certainly not scenic, for example. And, depending on your point of view, routes that cover the same lap more than once (the Blackpool marathon and Shakespeare marathon are both two laps, for example) can be helpful ... or soul-destroying.

# 15

# COUNTDOWN TO RACE DAY

## Tapering and race-day preparation

You could well be reading this section at a time when your marathon training is just beginning. But before you know it, all the hard weeks and months of preparation will be coming to an end.

It's natural to see race day as the crescendo of your training, but in reality, you'll have reached your peak training volume well before then, and will spend the final weeks gradually winding down. Marathon training takes its toll on the body, and this winding down period – the taper – enables important physiological adaptations to take place, microcellular damage to heal and accumulated fatigue to ease. In short, it allows you to consolidate the gains you've made (*see* 'Taper gains' on the next page). Studies show that when done properly, the controlled reduction in training load that the taper entails can yield a performance improvement of 2–4 per cent. For a four-hour marathoner, a 4 per cent improvement slices off 9 minutes and 36 seconds, bringing you over the line in 3 hrs 50 mins 24 secs.

When you think about it, it makes sense to take your foot off the pedal in the lead-up to race day. But instinctively, many people worry that they'll lose their fitness if they cut back on training, and end up disregarding the taper or throwing in panic-driven last-minute long runs. This is a big mistake, often resulting in you leaving your best performance out on the road *before* race day.

The fact is that many of the adaptations that have taken place in your body – such as increased capillarisation and mitochondria – are robust. They won't disappear overnight. A Danish study found that even four weeks of total inactivity didn't affect $VO_2$ max – and a well-executed taper certainly does not constitute total inactivity.

But it is worth making the point that the 'ideal' taper varies from person to person. Through trial and error, I've learned that a fairly strong three-week taper works best for me, but when I coached my husband for the Edinburgh marathon, a three-week taper left him feeling stale and he had a disappointing race. We've since learned that he responds better to a briefer period.

## TAPER GAINS

Will you really gain more by doing less? Let me count the ways…!

1. Improved running economy. A taper's effect on this important performance parameter is most prevalent among less experienced runners, according to a study in the journal *Sports Medicine*.

2. Restoration of immune function. Prolonged hard training suppresses the immune system and the taper helps reverse this, reducing the risk of infections.

3. Replenishment of glycogen stores in muscles and liver.

4. Improved levels of oxidative enzymes, which increases the rate at which energy can be produced aerobically.

5. More oxygen-carrying red blood cells. A two-week taper yielded an increase in red blood cells and haemoglobin concentration in a 2019 study.

6. Higher muscular power output. In a study on cross-country runners, a three-week taper led to increased power output, as a result of better fast-twitch muscle fibre function.

# Acing the taper caper

Whatever the length of the taper, the rules are the same. Rule number one (and this can sound counterintuitive) is that you don't cut out all the more challenging sessions and focus only on easy runs. Research has conclusively shown that maintaining some intensity within training (through race pace and tempo runs, threshold training and speedwork) is the single most important aspect of a successful taper.

In one 2019 study, runners performed no training slower than race pace during the taper. Some maintained a moderate volume while others tapered to a low volume. There was no significant difference in the results, demonstrating that intensity counted more than volume. In fact, the only study I found where the taper had a *negative* impact on performance (opposed to a positive one or no difference) was when intensity was reduced.

Just as you must maintain intensity, you must decrease volume. This is what lowers the overall training load. The scientific research suggests cutting back by 20–60 per cent of the peak volume that you reached in training. It's quite a wide range, and the right level for you will depend on how long you've been training, whether your training has been high-volume or not, how your body responds to training and your previous experiences of tapering. A study on Ethiopian runners found that training volume could be reduced by a whopping 70 per cent with no detrimental effects on performance. But these high-level athletes would have been sustaining a very high mileage in the first place. A 70 per cent reduction of 100 miles (160km) a week still leaves 30 miles (48.3km). A 70 per cent reduction of 30 miles (48.3km) a week leaves just 9 miles (14.5km). And indeed, a 2015 study from Loughborough University looking at the taper strategies of elite British runners found that a higher volume and frequency of training were associated with greater reductions in volume during the taper.

Sticking with the scientific research, it appears that decreasing volume is best achieved by reducing the *distance* of each run, and, in the case of your 'quality' sessions, reducing the quantity of reps or duration of efforts. Cutting down the number of times you run per week (frequency) is a less effective strategy – perhaps because the body likes routine and familiarity, or maybe because regular running maintains economy and neuromuscular efficiency. Or both.

You'll notice that no very long runs feature in the taper. At this late stage in the game, they are just not necessary – they will have zero impact on your fitness for race day, as there isn't enough time for the endurance adaptations to cement themselves. More likely, they will increase your fatigue and delay your recovery.

So far, we've only talked about running – if you're using cardiovascular cross-training activities in place of some runs, the same tapering rules outlined here apply. But I'd advise putting strength training aside in the last 7–10 days before the race to allow muscles to recover fully.

## Taper length

In the marathon programmes in this book, I've built in three-week tapers, which is the most commonly prescribed length for a marathon taper. But some people (like my husband, for instance) fare better with a two-week taper. If you have no prior marathon experience, it is probably best to err on the side of caution and go longer rather than shorter. But you can also factor in your response to long runs in training to help you determine how sharply to taper.

Marathon and ultrarunning blogger Jonathan Savage – better known as Fellrnr – has come up with a useful yardstick: if long runs leave you sore the next day – that is, you experience muscle pain on movement or palpation (pressing the muscle) – it's best to allow 21 days to taper. If long runs leave you fatigued (muscle weakness and a lower ability to exert force) but not sore, consider 14–21 days.

There's no need to do anything special diet-wise during the majority of your taper – continue to eat according to the guidelines in Chapter 17, being mindful that as your training winds down, your energy requirement will also drop a little. Over the final 24 hours, you might consider doing a carb load, which you can read more about on p. 209.

## Maranoid, me?

It's very common to experience some strange symptoms during the marathon taper. So common, in fact, that the term 'maranoia' has been invented to describe it. Heavy legs, aches and pains, symptoms of illness, feelings of anxiety and an unusually high RPE on runs are all frequently reported. Don't panic! One of the reasons you may feel 'heavier' than usual is because your glycogen stores are not being depleted as much by running – each gram of glycogen is stored with 3g of water. But fear not, this is dissipated as the glycogen is utilised. Another reason could be that, whether out of misguided intention or unknowingly, you're eating more (read more about race week fuelling on p. 209). But generally, these symptoms are all in the mind. Don't be tempted to 'boost your confidence' with an additional long run.

With less time spent running, you might find yourself with spare time on your hands. Try not to fill this time with extra socialising, tiring chores (like all that DIY or gardening you need to catch up on!) or, indeed, extra work. As discussed in Chapter 6, there's some evidence that mental fatigue can be detrimental to performance.

If you can wind down your mental workload – minimising stress and cognitive demands in the last couple of weeks before your race – do so. Consider it a 'mental taper', to add to your physical one.

## Planning your race strategy

While you are worrying about under-tapering, over-tapering and whether someone has poured concrete in your running shoes, here's something to take your mind off it.

Race-day preparation. We'll look at all the practical stuff in a moment, but first let's consider the race plan. How are you going to 'execute' your marathon? Are you thinking of using a pacer? Are you going to check your pace at every mile/km marker or run by feel? What's the fuelling strategy?

The first step is to determine your goal, which could be a specific time (3 hrs 29 mins) or a range (4 hrs 30 mins–4 hrs 45 mins). Many first-timers are nervous about having a time goal, but in my mind, having no idea of what you want to achieve risks starting out too fast and fading in the second half, or running overcautiously and not achieving what you're capable of.

We talked in Chapter 3 about figuring out your goal and it's worth revisiting this now that you have the bulk of your training behind you and race day is drawing closer. You will have new experience, fitness and knowledge about yourself as a runner, so factor this in as you reflect on what is realistic and achievable.

Race prediction calculators are a useful tool in this process, but also look closely at how you've responded to training. If, for example, you ran an 18-miler (29km) at 10-minute-miling (6 mins 12 secs per km) and felt shattered afterwards, is it realistic to expect to achieve 9-minute-miling (5 mins 35 secs per km) over an additional 8 miles (12.9km) on race day? Slowing your goal pace by 20–30 secs per mile (12.4–18.6 secs per km) will

make the race far more comfortable and your chances of success greater –
and this is particularly true if you are running your first marathon, when
your sense of pace over the distance will be less well honed.

Many sport psychologists recommend having multiple goals, rather
than a single target. For example, you might have a goal to cross the finish
line smiling, or to complete the race without hitting the wall. The theory
is that even if you don't make your goal time, you have other goals that can
still be achieved. Even within the realms of a goal time, you can broaden
things out by setting a bronze, silver and gold target. Bronze might simply
be completing the race, if you're a first-timer, silver could be doing so in
under 4 hrs 45 mins, and gold in under 4 hrs 35 mins.

## Doing the splits

Having a goal time – or goal time range – gives you an idea of what your
'splits' should be. (Splits are simply the amount of time it takes to run
any defined distance.) For the marathon, we're concerned mostly about
mile/kilometre splits and also first and second half splits of the entire
race. If you are aiming to run at an even pace, then your mile/km splits
won't differ significantly throughout the race. But some coaches – me
included – recommend a 'negative' split, whereby you plan to start out at
a slower pace and gradually speed up – meaning that the second half of
your race takes less time than the first half. Many of the best-ever times
run in marathons, including Eliud Kipchoge's 2018 official world record
and Paula Radcliffe's world record that stood for more than 16 years, were
achieved using a negative split.

The truth is, most runners end up running a positive split – where the
second half takes more time (often, a *lot* more time!) than the first, due to
a gradual slowing down over the course of the race. A study of more than
6000 participants of the Vienna Marathon found that every single one ran
a positive split.

You could use this as an argument for not bothering to try for a
negative split – hardly anyone manages it. But perhaps the reason they
don't is because they a) don't set off with a proper race strategy or b) are
targeting an unrealistic finish time, which leads to their pace dropping
off in the latter stages of the race.

I get it. The lure of going out hard and hanging on as long as you can
is strong. And you may even find that it's worked for you in other races.

But the marathon is different. Going out too fast means you burn through carbohydrates more quickly, raising the risk of hitting the wall.

My preference for road marathons is to aim for a modest negative split. This helps me avoid the all-too-common error of going off too fast and also reduces the stress of a crowded first few miles, when I might otherwise be panicking about 'losing' time. If that feels too daunting for you, then I definitely recommend aiming for even splits if your race route is flat, or an even effort level if it's a hilly course.

## Real-world pacing

Let's look at an example of how you might plan your pacing strategy.

Jane tells me she wants to run sub-4 hrs. Her half-marathon time of 1 hr 46 mins (achieved in a recent 'test' race, meaning it is a reliable indicator of her current fitness) suggests this is well within her capabilities (race prediction calculator estimates range from 3 hrs 42 mins to 3 hrs 56 mins) so we opt for a goal time of 3 hrs 56 mins, giving a little leeway for getting in under the four hours.

Jane could run 9-minute miles (5 mins 35 secs per km) throughout – 'even splits' – to achieve 3 hrs 56 mins. Or she could aim to run the first half of the race a little slower, at 9 mins 05 secs per mile (5 mins 38 secs per km), and the second half a little quicker (8 mins 55 secs per mile/5 mins 32 secs per km), which would theoretically bring her to the finish line at just under 3 hrs 56 mins. This would be a negative split, because if you divided the race in two, the second half would take less time than the first.

There's another form of negative splitting known as the 10-10-10 method, because the idea is to break the race distance down into three chunks: two 10-milers (16km) and one 10K (6.2 miles). You run the first 10-miler conservatively (with your head), the second 10-miler at your goal race pace (with your training) and the final 10K with your heart – no constraints! Why would you choose to do this? Well, by holding back just a little in the earlier stages, you might find that you have the energy to speed up significantly over those final miles.

Whichever protocol you use, deliberately setting off conservatively over the first 10–13 miles (16–21km) allows you to reach the halfway point still feeling good, raising the chances of a strong finish. This may be particularly worth considering if you are male – research suggests that men slow more significantly in the marathon than women.

## Safety in numbers?

Many marathons now provide pacers, who are enlisted to get runners across the finish line at key 'breakthrough' time points, from the magical sub-3 to sub-5 – and even 'just get round'. These pacers are generally experienced runners, assigned to get their group over the line using even pacing in a time that doesn't overstretch them personally, to maximise the chances of their success. You'll be able to find out in advance of race day whether pacers are going to be present at your target race and in what, and how many, pace ranges. Then you need to decide – will you run with them? I've run as a pacer at the London Marathon and I think there are pluses and minuses to consider.

One advantage is that it takes away some of the pressure of having to keep check on your watch all the time. It also provides a social element, with others to encourage and support you. But large groups around a pacer can be logistically difficult to stay with and you certainly don't want to be wasting energy ducking and diving in order to keep with them. Also, pacers are only human and there is no cast-iron guarantee that they'll get it right.

One of the crucial deciding factors is how close the pacer's target finish time is to your own. If, for example, you estimate that you are capable of finishing in 3 hrs 50 mins, I wouldn't advise running with the 3 hrs 45 mins pacer. Putting that extra time pressure on yourself in the early stages of the race might not feel significant, but later, when you're tired, it could come back and bite you. If you really want to run with a pace group, it'd be safer to run with the sub-4 hrs pacer for a good chunk of the race and then part ways with them later on, if you've got energy in the tank and want to press on for your goal time. There's no obligation to stay with a pacer, just because you started with them. But do say thank you and let them know you're off, if you can.

# Practical preparation for the race

## Course familiarisation

I am frequently amazed by how little research some runners do about their chosen race. For some, it's just a lack of organisation, for others it's a sort of nervous reaction – studying how far they've got to run is too daunting and they'd rather not think about it! But sometimes it is because a runner simply hasn't considered it might be helpful. It is.

Here a few things worth knowing:

- How many drinks stations are there and what will they have on offer?
- Is the course dead flat?
- Are there sections of rough ground or cobbles?
- Is it relatively straight or are there numerous twists and turns?
- What are the key landmarks?
- Is it a lap course or a single loop?

Race websites and entry packs will contain all this information and more. Don't leave finding out about the race until the last minute – acquaint yourself with it early in your training. It could even affect how you train – for example, a two-lap course might lead you to focus on 'half-and-half' long runs, in which you aim to run the second half a little faster than the first. If it's at all feasible, try to drive or cycle – or even run parts of – the route to familiarise yourself with it. The more acquainted you become with your course, the more you'll find your mind visualising running down the Champs-Elysées or along Brighton seafront or whatever.

Once you are into your Taper phase, read all the race information again – things that didn't seem relevant months before are now essential knowledge:

- Where do you pick up your race number or will it be sent to you?
- What time do you need to arrive?
- Where will the baggage store be?
- Does the race finish in the same place it starts?
- How do you meet up with friends and family afterwards?

## Accommodation and food

If you are travelling to your race on a package that includes accommodation and transport, that's two less things to worry about. Otherwise, you'll need to figure out your plans well in advance (especially if it is one of the major marathons attended by thousands of runners).

Here are some points to consider about accommodation:

- If you can be at home the night before the race, you'll have the advantage of total control over your meals – and get to sleep in your own bed. But can you do it without necessitating a ridiculously early start and stressful journey? If the answer is yes (like when my mum used to live opposite the first mile marker in the London marathon!), then great. But otherwise, consider booking a hotel or other accommodation near the race. Staying with friends or family is another option – but check out the considerations below even in this scenario.
- How close is it to the start (or finish)? In my experience, a hotel near the start line is worth its weight in gold. Race morning is stressful enough without adding lengthy travel into the equation. A finish-line venue also has its merits, though, as you will likely be exhausted by then and not relish having to use public transport.
- Will you be able to get breakfast? I've stayed at many hotels over the years (especially in Paris) where hotels won't serve breakfast early enough for marathon runners to eat pre-race. If that's the case, you'll need to take your own. If they do offer an early breakfast, check it'll be something that you're accustomed to having before a long run.
- Are there places to eat nearby in which you'll be able to get suitable simple carb-rich meals the day before? You should be able to check this out online.
- Is the accommodation quiet at night? The last thing you want is a rowdy stag party or live music going on downstairs or next door! I always take a sleep mask and ear plugs, just in case. And I ask for a morning alarm call as well as setting my phone and watch.

## Spectators

If you have friends and family coming to support you when you run the marathon, make sure they have done their homework, too. For example, if they are planning to go to multiple vantage points, how will they get from one to the other? If it's a mass-participation event with large crowds, which side of the road will they be on, so you can look out for them? Where will they meet you at or near the finish? Of course, you'll be part of all these discussions but make it clear that you don't want to be formulating plans at the last minute when your stress levels may already be high.

## What to wear

Race-day kit need not be anything special. In fact, saving something new to wear 'for best' is a mistake, since you can't be sure it won't ride up, fall down or chafe in all the wrong places. A dress rehearsal on one of your last long runs is a great opportunity to put all your proposed kit to the test, including things like socks and hydration packs. If you are running for a charity, make sure you get the branded race vest or T-shirt well in advance so you can try it out – in my experience, well-meaning charities don't always get it right in terms of materials, cut and size. If the top isn't 100 per cent comfortable, you could offer to wear it for a photo at the start and finish and choose your own top for the race itself.

Of course, the best-laid plans can be thrown by changes in the weather. It's a good idea to have contingencies for different weather situations. I remember frantically cutting my running tights off above the knee one London Marathon race morning when the forecast suddenly shifted from weeks of grey chilly days to blazing sunshine, while Boston marathon participants in the spring of 2018 faced freezing temperatures, torrential rain and winds gusting at up to 45mph (70kph).

You can't control or even necessarily predict the weather but you can be prepared for every eventuality. One of the oldest – but best – pieces of advice you'll ever hear about race day is to take some old clothes with you that you're happy to part with. These will keep you warm after you've deposited your bag and can be discarded just before the gun goes. The ubiquitous bin liner, with arms and head hole cut out, is another must, keeping off rain as well as conserving body heat. You can read more about running in the heat – and other challenging weather – in Chapter 5.

Lots of people like to run wearing earphones but I would really discourage you from doing this in the race. (Indeed, some races don't allow them.) You'll miss out on the atmosphere of the day and the energy that spectators and other runners give out. If you're not convinced, why not try going 'naked' at a shorter race to see how you find it? Ultimately, you must do what feels right to you, but I always feel a bit sad when I see someone running among a crowd closed off in their own little world.

# Kit checklist

THERE IS NO definitive list of what to pack for your race – one runner's race-day essentials are another's idea of excess baggage. Other than my racing kit, my absolute essential is a pair of fresh socks and sandals to put on – not my most stylish look, but luxury for my battered feet! Here's what else to consider putting on your list:

- Race-day instructions;
- Race number;
- Safety pins, clips or a race belt to attach the race number to your top;
- Timing chip;
- Running shoes (read more about footwear in Chapter 7);
- Running socks;
- Calf guards;
- Comfortable underwear;
- Sports bra for women/nipple guards for men;
- Shorts or bottoms. I always go for a pair with a pocket, in which I'll carry some loo paper and a £20 note in case of emergency;
- Vest or T-shirt;
- Waterproof jacket. I've never run a marathon in a waterproof jacket, but if the weather is particularly bad, or if you envisage that you'll be out on the course for a very long time, then give it some thought;
- Hair band or ties to keep hair off your face;
- Sunglasses. These are worth considering even if it's not bright sunshine. They keep out grit and flies;
- Sunscreen and lip balm;
- Headphones (ideally, just for pre-race);
- Anti-chafe lube (for anywhere you might experience rubbing);
- Drinks bottle, belt or hydration pack, if using;
- Energy gels or other snacks. (Remember to include what you might want *before* the race, as well as your race fuel.);
- Old clothing to wear over race kit on race morning. Make sure it's easy to get off. Hat and gloves that you don't mind saying farewell to if you feel too warm. Bear in mind that you will be discarding your pre-race kit and won't have it for afterwards, so you'll also need to pack something to change into afterwards, including that comfortable footwear;
- Bin liner (or disposable mac).

# Eating your way through the last 24 hours

The days of lengthy and complex carbo-loading strategies are over – but research does support the use of a simple 24-hour carb load as a way of topping up those glycogen stores.

The aim is to consume 10g of carbohydrate/kg of your bodyweight (10g/2.2lb) over this period (starting with breakfast the day before the race) to achieve 'glycogen supercompensation'. To do this without increasing the overall amount of food that you eat, keep protein, fat and fibre to a minimum and focus on simple carbohydrate sources. The kind of foods that are usually best avoided, such as white bread and pasta, white rice, refined breakfast cereal, sugary juices and sweets are now the order of the day – but do ensure you are not inadvertently loading up with fat, in the form of pizza, pastry, chips and cakes! Conversely, the foods that we normally consider healthy, such as lean proteins, healthy oils and fats, wholegrains, green veg, beans and pulses, are not necessary during this short period, as they are unlikely to sit well on race day.

One of the good things about doing a 24-hour carb load is that it takes the emphasis off that 'last supper' – the much-heralded 'pasta fest' the night before the race. Instead, you are spreading your carbohydrate intake over a number of meals.

I like to eat my final pre-race dinner in the early evening, so that I don't end up going to bed feeling too full. If I get peckish later, I'll have a carb-rich snack.

I strongly recommend that you don't do a carb load for the first time just before your big day. If you're planning on doing it, practise it – ideally before a race, like a half-marathon, or before one of your longest long runs. In fact, whether you are carb loading or not, a 'meal rehearsal' – during which you eat all the exact meals you've got planned for this final 24-hour period before completing a race or run – is really worthwhile, so you can be confident that it all goes down well and doesn't cause any bloating, gas or other stomach trouble.

## Race morning

Allow plenty of time on race morning to prepare, eat and digest your final meal. Research suggests that two to four hours is the optimal amount of time between eating and running. But again, this is something you'll want to determine for yourself well before race day, through trial and error.

Whether you are doing the carb load or not, breakfast should be carb-focused, with little protein, fat or fibre. Sports nutritionists recommend that your marathon breakfast includes 1–4g of carbohydrate/kg of your bodyweight (1–4g/2.2lb). Examples might include toast and jam, porridge and honey, a bagel with banana or cornflakes and milk.

Even if you don't feel like eating, it is important to get some calories in. The mere act of sleeping for eight hours will have burned up liver glycogen and you want your energy stores to be fully loaded. Try an energy drink or meal replacement drink if you can't face solid foods.

Another important reason to eat in the morning is that it triggers the 'gastrocolic reflex', essentially stimulating a bowel movement. (Running on an empty stomach will not minimise the risk of a mid-race pit-stop.) The other thing that wakes up the bowels is movement – so allow time after eating your breakfast to potter around until you are ready to visit the loo. Coffee is another useful tool for getting you to 'go', because it contains compounds (alongside caffeine) that increase your body's levels of gastrin and cholecystokinin, hormones that increase colon activity.

Having eaten and visited the toilet, you're ready to pick up your kitbag and make your way to the start.

# 16
# MAKING RACE DAY A SUCCESS

## From start line to finish line ... and beyond

Arrive at the start area in good time but try to avoid getting there so early that you have hours in which to get cold, bored or nervous! Do the essential tasks – acquainting yourself with the start line (and the location of your 'pen' if the race is set up this way), dropping off your bag, queuing for the loo – and then try to relax until it is time to line up. The odd sip of sports drink or water is fine during this waiting period, but one of the best pieces of advice I can offer is to stop drinking in earnest one hour before the race. Since I started doing this, I have succeeded in restricting myself to one pre-race loo visit, rather than two or even three! And I've never needed to stop for a mid-race wee, either.

One of the issues with having a drink on hand right up until the race starts is that you tend to drink mindlessly, and by the time you're on the move, you're already wondering where the nearest Portaloo will be. Following the one-hour cut-off guideline allows your body time to absorb the fluid that you have consumed since waking up, get rid of the excess well before the gun goes and set off with an empty bladder. Once you begin running, blood will be diverted to your working muscles, rather than your kidneys, and it's unlikely that you'll be troubled by your bladder again.

If you are planning on taking caffeine, your last drink (approximately an hour before race start time) is a good time to do it as you can wash your caffeinated gel/sweets or caffeine pills down with some fluid and allow time for the caffeine to reach its peak in your bloodstream.

## Do I need to warm up?

Whether – and to what extent – you warm up is dependent on how fast you'll be running, relative to what feels comfortable to you. As I've explained, a faster runner isn't just running quicker than a slower runner, they're almost certainly running at a higher percentage of their own personal capacity than the slower runner (simply because a slower runner is less able to maintain a very high percentage of their maximum capacity for such a long duration).

If you're going to be running at a pace that feels somewhat challenging to you, you'll need to spend more time warming up than someone who will be sticking well within their comfort zone. But even then, the warm-up can be quite short and low-key, perhaps finishing with a few strides. Remember to stick to familiar routines – don't use race day to suddenly throw in Sun Salutations or pogo jumps if you don't usually. You might find that the time you need to enter the start pen simply doesn't allow you the space and time to warm up as you would wish. If this is the case, don't worry too much. You can do some mobility work on the spot and use your opening miles to gradually ease into your desired pace.

## The marathon morning mindset

It's natural to feel nervous on race day. It's because this marathon *means something* to you and it certainly isn't a sign that anything is wrong. But if you do have butterflies, you want them to be flying in formation. Avoiding last-minute stress by being super-organised helps to dispel anxiety and uncertainty (*see* 'Practical preparation for the race' on p. 204). But there are some other useful strategies to get your head in the right place.

### Find your zone

You only need to watch the line-up at any athletics event on TV to see that some competitors are bristling and bouncing with nervous energy while others appear calm and even distant. Sports psychologists talk about something called the 'zone of optimal functioning' – which is the pre-performance mental state that is most conducive to a competitor's ability to perform at their best. It usually falls somewhere around the middle of a continuum on which completely laid-back and relaxed is on one end and intensely psyched-up is on the other. But the sweet spot is different for everyone. You might have found that you get quite hyper pre-race, chatting to other runners, snapping selfies and double- and triple-checking your kit – or that you prefer to sit quietly with headphones on, keeping out of the melee.

If you are not sure, think back to previous race experiences (and other stressful life experiences) to get an idea of what works best for you – and then make sure that you honour that. Your family or colleagues might be coming along to support you and want to ask you lots of questions about the race and take photos, but if you'd rather be on your own to gather your thoughts, tell them so.

## And breathe

Focusing on your breath is a tried-and-tested way of calming pre-performance anxiety. The mere act of focusing your attention on it tends to bring it under control. Slow your inhalation by counting to four as you breathe in; then exhale for a count of six. Let your lower ribcage expand and your abdomen relax as you inhale, rather than lifting your shoulders and chest.

## Mind what you say

'I bet I hit the wall.' 'I'm never going to get round without walking.' 'My dodgy knee is sure to flare up...' You might not think it matters all that much what you say to yourself, but science suggests otherwise. Negative 'self-talk' can have a profound effect on your self-esteem and confidence, and even affect the way you behave. For example, if you are convinced that you're going to hit the wall, you might disregard your pre-planned pacing strategy and just try to get as far as you can before fatigue catches up with you – sabotaging your whole race. In fact, one study, published in the *Journal of Sports and Exercise*, found that people who expected to hit the wall were more likely to!

Having a phrase or two that you can repeat to yourself when negative thoughts come in can be helpful. Known as a mantra, this phrase should be short, meaningful and comprise positive words. So 'I am not a loser' doesn't pass muster.

## Dispel fear and anxiety

The other thing that can help with negative thinking is something psychologists call 'if-then' planning. This strategy allows you to address your worries in a practical way. The idea is to identify the things you are anxious about happening (such as it being really hot on race day, needing the toilet or getting a blister) and work out a contingency plan for what you will do in that event. You cannot control everything. If it's pouring with rain on race morning, there's nothing you can do to change that. But you can be more prepared to deal with it (for example, taking a bin liner or rain mac to the start, which you can discard once you begin running.) You can also remind yourself that you have run in the rain on many previous occasions and that once you get going, you'll barely notice it.

Here's an example: *if* I need a wee on the start line ... *then* I will wait until I've started running, as it could just be nerves. If the feeling doesn't go away after the first couple of miles, I will take a pit-stop. (Of course, if you follow the advice to stop drinking an hour before the race start, it is far less likely that this particular problem will arise!)

My final tip is to use a neurolinguistic programming (NLP) technique called the 'Circle of Excellence'. This is a way of 'gathering together' all the attributes you're going to need to run a successful marathon. Imagine a circle – big enough to stand in – on the ground, or draw a real one. Stand next to it and think of a quality you'll need. For example, determination. Recall an occasion in your life when you showed real determination. What did it feel like? Use all your senses to recreate that sense of pushing through, no matter how many obstacles stood in your way. Once you can really feel it, step into the circle and 'deposit' determination there. Step back out and repeat this process with the other attributes you want – confidence, focus, control... When all your desired resources are inside your circle, step away and pick it up. You might want to imagine that you're putting it into your pocket or tucking it under your watch strap, where it will be ready and waiting for you to 'unpack' and step into just before the race.

# On your marks...

There's an old saying about the marathon that I think does a good job of highlighting how it's the training that precedes it that is the true challenge. It goes: 'A marathon is hundreds of miles. The last 26.2 miles is the finish.' Well, you've reached the last 26.2 miles (42.2km) – so let's make sure all your hard work is put to good use.

The start pen of a major city marathon can be an intense place. (Read more about race selection in Chapter 14.) The proximity of bodies, the clamour of noise, the smell of muscle rub! Do what you need to do to stay within your zone of optimal functioning, be that calm or excited. If you are running with a pacer, make your way over to them.

Check your shoelaces are secure. If there's space, you could adopt a 'power stance' – legs a bit wider than hip distance apart, upright posture, chest up, hands on hips – if you dare! Research has shown that this 'dominant' pose helps to boost confidence, lowering levels of cortisol (the stress hormone) and boosting testosterone.

A few minutes before the off, discard any clothing you don't want to run in and take your first energy gel or snack. You'll be running by the time the carbs it contains enter your bloodstream, but you'll have avoided the faff of consuming it on the move and reduced the risk of GI distress. The only scenario in which you wouldn't do this would be if you took a caffeinated energy gel an hour before the start, which will have already topped up your glucose levels.

And finally ... after all the weeks and months of preparation, you are off!

## Running the race

Let's start with one of those pieces of advice that is given so often it sounds almost too obvious. *Do not go off too fast*. Research has shown that when marathon runners begin the race at a pace that is just 2 per cent quicker than their practised goal pace, they flounder over the final 6 miles (10km). The reason this advice is so often repeated is because it is so rarely heeded. It is probably the most common marathon mistake that runners make. Embarrassing as it is to admit, I even did it myself not so long ago. I'd had a break from marathon running and decided I'd do one to celebrate my 50th birthday. My goal pace was 8-minute-miling (4 mins 58 secs per km), but after my taper, I was feeling good and found myself going through the first 2 miles (3.2km) closer to 7 mins 45 secs per mile (4 mins 48 secs per km) pace. 'Ah well,' I thought. 'I'm probably in better shape than I thought...' I kept the faster pace going for around 10 miles (16km), hit goal pace for a further 6–7 miles (10–11km) and then fell into a sharp decline. I ended up finishing 15 minutes slower than I'd planned to. Don't do the same! You have a goal pace and a race plan, so use them.

That said, you don't want to be checking your pace every few seconds. That way lies madness and quite possibly, a tumble as you trip over another runner's feet or discarded bin bag or bottle. I tend to glance at my watch two or three times in the opening mile or two and after that, generally only at mile markers. But if you're not confident of your ability to 'sense' your pace, then you may want to look a little more often.

In one of my best marathon performances, I chatted to a fellow runner for the first 4 miles (6.4km). I'm quite a solitary runner most of the time, so this wasn't usual for me – but it meant that I ran at a relaxed pace in those early, nervous miles and it put me in a positive mindset, both of which helped my race.

## IS DRAFTING WORTH IT?

The energy cost of overcoming wind resistance on a calm day is 2 per cent for a runner at a pace of 5 mins 30 secs per mile (3 mins 25 secs per km). At faster paces, the cost is higher. But given that most of us won't be hitting the heady heights of a sub 2 hrs 30 mins marathon, is overcoming wind resistance an issue? On a calm day, not really. But if there's a strong headwind, the energy cost will be much greater and you may benefit from tucking in behind another runner. Research suggests that you need to be no less than 1m (3.3ft) behind the runner in front to benefit – which is pretty close. So if you do decide that drafting could be worthwhile, it's probably best to ask another runner or small group if they want to take turns at the front rather than sneaking in behind someone and risking clipping each other's feet. Also ensure that you are as aerodynamic as possible in terms of your kit (not flappy) and hair (tied back, slicked down or contained under a cap or hat).

At the front of the pack, running with others is less about socialising and more about performance. Having people to stick with, and possibly draft off, can really help you get the best out of yourself. For most of us non-elites, the chances are there'll be so many other people around that there'll be no opportunity – or need – for drafting. But running with another runner or a small group can still be mentally beneficial.

While the marathon is quite evidently 26.2 miles or 42.2km – it is best to break the distance down into more digestible chunks in your head once you are actually running. This could be done using landmarks on the course, or with specific distances (like the 10-10-10 method I described on p. 203).

I say the marathon is 26.2 miles (42.2km), but in many of the major city marathons, people often find themselves running significantly further, due to having to weave between other runners as they make their way along the course. If you start in the right pen for your speed and don't panic in the early miles you can minimise this energy-sapping movement. You'll also reduce your risk of tripping or collisions if you hold your course.

On a hot day, it's worth sticking to the shadier, cooler parts of the course where possible, to reduce the impact on your performance. It's also a smart move to pour water over your head at regular intervals to help you feel cooler. In one study, a group of runners endured 33°C (91.4°F) heat while they ran 5K time trials. Spraying cold water on their faces lowered their forehead temperature and 'thermal sensation' (how hot they felt). Read more about running in the heat in Chapter 5.

## Overcoming obstacles – and the W-word

One of the things I tell the runners I coach is that they will almost certainly go through a bad patch during the marathon. They always look worried or disappointed when I say this, but I think it's actually a really positive thing to go into the race with the knowledge that at some point, it's going to be tough and you're going to have to summon up hitherto untapped resources of strength and determination. When that bad patch comes along, you can just think 'Ah, here's that bad patch. It'll pass' while ensuring that you take all the steps possible to make it pass quickly. (*See* 'Dropping out' for advice on what to do if it doesn't.)

# DROPPING OUT

There are times in a marathon when the thought of dropping out might pop into your head. This is a tough physical and mental challenge, and you aren't necessarily going to be smiling the whole way round. If it's general fatigue, rather than a specific problem, such as a painful tendon, that's putting you off, dig deep into your mental and physical reserves to keep going (see 'Race-day tactics' on p. 219). If, however, you feel incapable of making it to the finish, and believe that to try to do so would be detrimental to your health, it is wise to live to fight another day, rather than push yourself beyond your limits and end up ill or badly injured. **If you suffer from repeated diarrhoea or vomiting on the way round, feel dizzy or faint, or experience chest pain accompanied by severe breathlessness, please stop at an aid station and seek medical assistance.**

Dropping out of a marathon is a difficult decision to make – months of training and hard work, possibly with the added burden of fundraising, are inevitably big incentives to continue, but you must heed your body's warning signs if you are feeling unwell or are in pain.

If you do decide to pull out, make sure you let a marshal or first aid station know. They should be able to advise you on how to get back to the finish area (or start) if you're able to do so and/or notify the race organisers or your friends and family. Some marathons arrange buses to help runners who have had to drop out, but this isn't always possible at events where there are fewer runners and miles of open roads. This is when that bankcard or cash in your shorts pocket may prove invaluable.

Go through the basics: do you need a drink or a gel? Is your pace appropriate? Are you as relaxed as possible? Can you cheer yourself up by interacting with spectators, taking in the sights around you, speaking to another runner? It could be that you're experiencing a motivational malfunction. Remind yourself why you are running this race. Congratulate yourself for all the hard work you have put in. Think how good it will feel to cross the line and how you'll be able to go to bed that night with a marathon (or another marathon) under your belt. And in the meantime, no matter how near or far away the finish line is, run the mile you're in. Then the next one.

A bad patch is not the same as hitting the wall. While a brief period of feeling sorry for yourself is almost inevitable, hitting the wall is not.

The wall is all to do with energy utilisation. You'll remember that the amount of glycogen you can store in the muscles and liver is limited. One of the key objectives of training is to make your body more efficient at using fat as a fuel source so that you can eke out your glycogen stores a bit longer. Another objective is to make your body ramp up its capacity for storing glycogen. Your training has equipped you to utilise energy efficiently and thereby avoid the wall. But if you run at a pace that is faster than the one you've trained for, you'll be eating into those glycogen stores from the off and will deplete them before you reach the finish line. Then your body needs to rely on fat. While you'd think that wouldn't be a problem (we carry enough body fat to fuel several marathons) the breakdown of fat for fuel takes place at a lower intensity, forcing you to slow down. Often, dehydration plays a role in hitting the wall, too.

The first port of call if you feel yourself crashing is to address fuel and hydration intake, using the guidelines from Chapters 17 and 18. If you are using caffeine in your nutrition plan, now would be a good time to take a booster dose. Keep moving at whatever pace you can, and if you've responded quickly enough to the situation, you'll likely find your way out the other side.

# 7 race–day tactics

### 1. Turn that frown upside down

Smiling makes running feel easier. Sounds like nonsense? Not according to Eliud Kipchoge, the sub-2-hr-marathon world record holder. After his world first performance, he explained that he smiled intermittently to help himself relax and ignore the pain of such intense effort. There's evidence to back this up. The 'facial feedback theory' suggests that just as hard efforts cause us to frown, intentional frowning makes us perceive what we're doing as hard. Researchers at Ulster University monitored runners while they smiled or frowned and found that running economy was 2 per cent better when smiling. Their rate of perceived exertion was also lower. News to get you grinning like the Cheshire cat...

## 2.  Dedicate each mile

People often talk about running with your heart, and this – an idea I first heard from a lovely runner called Joan whom I knew many years ago – is a great way of really making that resonate. When you are running each mile of the race for a particular person that you care about, every single mile is meaningful. I applied this strategy to a 12-hour cycling time trial once, attributing each hour I rode to a different person. I spent that hour thinking of all the happy memories I had of that person. It worked a treat.

## 3.  Body scan

Plan to run through a body scan (see p. 156) at regular intervals throughout the race. For example, just after you've taken on a gel or passed a mile marker. Start at your feet and make your way up to your head, 'checking in' to ensure that you are maintaining good form and posture and staying relaxed. Common sites for tension include the neck and shoulders, jaw, hands and ankles.

## 4.  Play to the crowd

Studies show that we perform better when we are being watched. Research conducted at John Hopkins University in 2018 found that when people playing a video game were watched, they performed 5 per cent better than when they had no audience. One way of tapping into this so-called 'audience effect' is to engage with the crowd. Get your head up and make eye contact with spectators. Listen to their words of encouragement and applause. It is for you!

## 5.  Take your mind off it

When you are struggling with discomfort or fatigue, try to distract yourself. Counting to 500 was Paula Radcliffe's favoured tactic – she knew it would roughly equate to another mile run. Try guessing what gel flavour you're going to pull out next, or what colour your next jelly sweet will be. Read the funny signs that people hold up.

### 6.  Talk nicely to yourself

Some research published in the *Journal of Personality and Social Psychology* found that talking to yourself using the word 'you' rather than 'I' could be more effective. I've found that I spontaneously do this – saying to myself (not out loud) 'well done, you're doing really well'. Imagining someone you respect or care about – such as your coach or partner – saying the words can also be powerful. And remember your mantras. I like 'easy, light, smooth' and 'just keep going'.

### 7.  Use other runners

Once you are into the final miles, pick a runner who is a little way ahead of you. Imagine that you are being drawn towards them by a magnet, or hauling yourself closer with a rope. Alternatively, see if you can match their cadence – you'll almost certainly find that your pace picks up. Even if you don't manage to catch anyone up, these tactics give you something to focus on.

## The finish line

No matter how tired you are, you will probably discover a 'second wind' when you see the finish line ahead. This demonstrates how much running is a mental battle as well as a physical one, as discussed in Chapter 6. Finish as strongly as you can and regardless of how the race has gone in relation to your hopes and expectations, smile. You will have done the best you could on the day and you're a bloody hero. Remember that.

## Post-race survival

Try to keep moving once you cross the line, rather than stopping suddenly. As soon as you are able to, eat and drink something, ideally something that fits the bill in terms of carbohydrate and protein intake. As a reminder, the perfect recovery prescription consists of carbohydrate – around 1g of carbohydrate/kg of your bodyweight (1g/2.2lb) – along with 0.25–0.3g protein/kg of bodyweight (0.25–0.3g/2.2lb). I often take a carton of chocolate milk in my kitbag for immediate post-race refuelling.

Change into dry, comfortable kit. If you have a long journey home, try to break it up with short periods of standing up and walking around to avoid getting even stiffer. Forgo static stretching – your muscles are likely to be sore and inflamed, and it's better to just let them recover for a day or two. Sip fluids regularly for the remainder of the day, being mindful of thirst and frequency (and colour) of urination.

There are two things that I try to do post-marathon that I find helpful. One is to get into water (I say that rather than 'swim' as it's more a case of floating around than actual swimming!). Being buoyant takes the weight off the joints and the hydrostatic pressure (the pressure of the water against your body) aids venous return as well as easing swelling and muscle pain. A study in the *International Journal of Sports Medicine* found that a swimming-based recovery session after running enhanced exercise performance the next day, compared to passive recovery. Not that I'm suggesting you should run the day after your marathon...

My other routine procedure post-marathon is to wear a pair of compression tights for a few hours. While the science on their efficacy is mixed (read more in Chapter 9), I feel more comfortable with them on, even if they aren't actually serving a physiological purpose. I also admit I'm quite a fan of an afternoon nap following a morning marathon, followed by a gentle walk and dinner. A meal that is rich in omega-3s and antioxidants is a good choice, as these nutrients help dampen inflammation. Oily fish with vegetables and rice or potatoes would fit the bill perfectly. But if you fancy a blowout curry or a giant pizza, go for it. You deserve it.

In addition to your immediate refuelling (as soon as possible after finishing running), be vigilant about consuming 20–40g (⅔–1⅓oz) of protein at subsequent meals and snacks. Aim for 1.2–1.8g of protein/kg of your bodyweight (1.2–1.8g/2.2lb) over the course of each day for the following 72 hours. Research in the journal *Nutrients* found that making use of this prolonged post-exercise recovery window was beneficial in hastening recovery.

## Recovering from the marathon

The level of stress that your body experiences running a marathon has a significant effect on the immune system. Indeed, studies show that immune function is compromised for up to three days.

You'll also be feeling stiff and sore, particularly in the couple of days following the race when DOMS is likely to peak. The best way to assist recovery is to include small amounts of gentle activity each day, get plenty of rest and be diligent about protein intake. Revisit the section on recovery for a reminder of some of the most helpful practices (*see* p. 145).

I recommend not running for a full week. I know many runners do, but studies show that people who rest for a whole week actually fare better in subsequent training than do those who attempt to run in the first few days. The body needs this time to replenish energy stores, repair muscle damage and allow minor afflictions, such as chafing and blisters, to heal. It also gives you a mental break and enables you to re-attune to 'normal' life. If you feel up to it, you might do some gentle non-running activity during this week – such as swimming or Pilates. A few days post-race is also the best time to schedule a sports massage.

Don't feel you *have* to get back to running after a week off. If you want longer, then take it. And don't be surprised if, when you do get back to running, you don't immediately feel as fit as you did pre-marathon. A good way to ease back in is with a reverse taper. Just as you wound down your training as the race drew closer, you gradually increase the volume of training in the post-race weeks to a level that you're happy with. (Which doesn't, incidentally, mean you have to get back to your marathon-training volume.)

## Reflect and review

It's quite common to feel a sense of anticlimax once the race is over. This has been a huge part of your life for months and now it's done, there's a big empty space. Knowing this might happen can lessen the impact of such an unexpected feeling. Making sure you have something planned a few days after the race that you're really looking forward to will give you something positive to focus on.

But don't leave it too long to reflect on how your race went – do it while it's still fresh in your mind. Whether you achieved your goal or not, pinpoint what you did well and what you could have done better. Did your choice of kit work out well? Did you get your hydration right? If you could train for the marathon again, what would you do differently and why? This is all valuable information about yourself as a runner that will feed into future performances. There is no need to put another race in the diary straight away. You may choose to just enjoy running with no set rules and time goals for a while. But if you're like most marathon runners, you'll soon find yourself back on the start line.

# NUTRITION AND HYDRATION

# 17
# FUEL FOR THOUGHT

## Nutrition for health, performance and recovery

In my experience, many runners put a lot of thought and effort into their training but very little into ensuring they eat and drink the right things to support it. Yet good nutrition is key for optimal health, performance and recovery.

What do I mean by 'good nutrition'? A healthy, balanced diet that provides a wide range of nutrients and sufficient energy (calories) for your needs. I'm certainly not saying that chips and cake should be off-limits – everyone needs to indulge now and then – but when you're putting your body through the rigours of marathon training, the right nutritional support is more important than ever. Even if you've 'got by' so far without giving what you eat a second thought, I'd urge you to think more carefully about your nutrition in the weeks and months leading up to your marathon.

### Meeting your energy needs

The basics for a marathon-training diet are the same as for any healthy diet. But there are two key factors to consider. First, quantity – you'll need to ensure your calorie intake matches your increased energy expenditure. And second, timing – what nutrients you eat when for maximum benefit.

A broad guideline for the energy cost of running is 62 calories per km (100 calories per mile/1.6km). (*See* 'Estimating your energy expenditure' below for a more accurate method.) So, if your weekly distance increases from, say, 20 miles (32km) per week to 30 miles (48km) per week, you'll be burning around 1000 additional calories. To maintain a stable bodyweight, you would need to up your calorie intake by that amount. (In our example, that would mean consuming an additional 140 calories per day: 7 x 140 = 980.) However, if you're carrying excess baggage as you embark on your marathon training and would like to shed a couple of kilograms or pounds, keeping your energy intake constant as weekly distance climbs will create a deficit (in our example, a modest deficit of 1000 calories per week). That way, you will gradually shed weight over the course of your marathon training without needing to actively *cut* calories. But monitor your weight (use scales if you like, or check how your clothing fits) and energy levels as you go, to ensure that you don't end up under-fuelling in pursuit of weight loss. Failing to meet your energy needs will be counterproductive, either leading you to skip sessions because of fatigue or push through them and risk injury.

## Estimating your running energy expenditure

MULTIPLY THE NUMBER of kilometres you run by your bodyweight (in kg) to get your approximate energy expenditure in calories.
Example. You run 5km and you weigh 70kg. 5 x 70 = 350 calories.

The food and drink you consume provides the energy you need for every bodily function, from breathing, digesting and thinking to walking and running. The 'big three' providers are known as the macronutrients: 1) carbohydrates (which provide 4 calories per gram), 2) proteins (4 calories per gram) and 3) fats (9 calories per gram).

Food also provides vitamins and minerals (micronutrients), which don't contain energy in the form of calories, but are essential to good health and bodily function (including hormonal, metabolic and immune function). Plant foods have an added bonus, in the form of health-giving compounds called phytonutrients, such as lycopene in tomatoes, resveratrol in grapes and quercetin in onions. Every nutrient has a unique role and value, which is why a varied diet is so important, not to mention more interesting and satisfying in terms of flavours and textures.

## Carbohydrates are king

So where should these extra calories to fuel your marathon training come from? Carbohydrates are the body's preferred source of energy for anything other than the lightest exercise intensity, as well as being the only fuel source the brain can use.

The carbs you consume are converted to glucose, and transported in the bloodstream for storage as glycogen in the muscles (typically 300–400g/10½–14oz) and liver (80–100g/2¾–3½oz) – providing 1520–2000 calories worth of energy. Physical activity will deplete levels, as will insufficient calorie intake (which triggers the body to convert some of its glycogen back into glucose). That's why it is so important to make carbs a regular feature of your marathon-training diet.

As a runner, at least 50 per cent of your overall calorie intake should be coming from carbohydrates; but a more useful and specific goal to strive for is around 5–6g carbs/kg of your bodyweight (5–6g/2.2lb). You may have read recommendations considerably higher than this – as high as 8–12g/kg (8–12g/2.2lb) but these figures are based on the needs of elite athletes, who are training at much higher volumes than most of us, and consuming a lot more calories overall. If your training load is moderate – say, four to six hours a week – then 5–6g/kg is a good aim, at least to begin with. You can always adjust up or down when you know how your body is responding. It's only when you're training for two or more hours a day every day that you'd consider taking on 8–10g/kg (8–10g/2.2lb) of carbohydrate routinely. If we take a 70kg (11 stone) runner as an example, you'll see why: if they were to consume 10g/kg (10g/2.2lb) that would be 700g (1½lb) of carbohydrate per day. Given that each gram of carbohydrate contains 4 calories, that would mean (4 x 700) 2800 calories coming from carbohydrates alone, before they've even considered protein or fat intake. You'd need to be training exceedingly hard to require this number of calories – and any excess will, of course, be converted to body fat. The only other scenario in which you might turbocharge your carb intake to this degree is during a pre-race 'carbo-load', that you can read about on p. 209.

All that said, it would seem that many runners *are* falling short on carbohydrate. A 2016 study found that less than half consumed sufficient carbohydrate, based on sports nutrition recommendations, while 87 per cent met protein guidelines. Meeting your carbohydrate needs is particularly important during periods of intensified training – such as building up to a marathon. A study at Birmingham University found that when additional training demands were placed on a group of runners, a high-carbohydrate intake (65 per cent of total calorie intake) helped them tolerate this more successfully than did a lower intake (41 per cent). While the high-carb diet enabled runners to maintain their performance in a 10-mile (16km) time trial, the low-carb diet group saw a gradual worsening of performance.

Here are some of the best sources of healthy carbs in your daily diet:

- Wholegrains (oats, wholemeal flour, brown rice, quinoa, bulgar wheat, barley, wholewheat pasta);
- Pulses (beans, peas and lentils);
- Starchy veg (potatoes/sweet potato, squash, carrots, beetroot, sweetcorn). These also pack a nutrient-fuelled punch, being rich in fibre, B vitamins, iron and magnesium.

*See* the table in Appendix 1 on p. 275 for the carbohydrate content of some common foods to see how you can build a carbohydrate-rich diet that will support your running.

One final sell for carbohydrates: they support the immune system, reducing the risk of those frustrating interruptions to training due to coughs, colds and other infections. One study found that consuming a low-carbohydrate diet (30 per cent of total energy intake) led to higher markers of immune stress during three days of intense training compared to a high-carbohydrate diet (60 per cent of the total). Another found that consuming up to 60g (2oz) of carbohydrate during intense exercise (which we'll look at later in this section) helped to attenuate the immune inflammatory response.

## Protein intake

While the bulk of your additional calories should come from carbohydrate, you may also need a little more protein than usual during marathon training, to assist in muscle repair and growth. A good guideline for runners regarding protein intake is 1.2–1.8g/kg of bodyweight (1.2–1.8g/2.2lb) per day. There are three groups of people who may need to look towards the higher end of this range:

1.  Runners venturing into the territory of this level of training for the first time (who are less efficient at consolidating protein into their muscles);
2.  Runners undertaking a very high volume of training (more training = more muscle damage);
3.  Runners aged 50+ (a greater intake of protein is required to stimulate muscle protein synthesis among older runners).

However, protein deficiency is rare in the Western diet – rather than unthinkingly upping your protein intake, it's worth trying to figure out how much you currently consume. As the research mentioned above found, it's much more likely that you are under-consuming carbohydrate than protein. The protein content chart in Appendix 1 on p. 276 will help.

Protein is best consumed in frequent small doses – 20–40g (⅔–1⅓oz) at a time – rather than attempting to 'load' it into one meal. Research shows that this is the most efficient way to maximise muscle protein synthesis, support performance and maintain a healthy body composition.

Good protein sources include:

•   Lean meat, fish and seafood, eggs, dairy foods. These contain all eight 'essential' amino acids that you require from diet.
•   Legumes, grains, nuts and seeds. Plant proteins contain fewer essential amino acids or in a less favourable ratio than animal-derived sources. Combining a grain with a pulse, nut or seed offers the complete set of essential amino acids – for example, hummus and pitta, rice and beans, wholemeal bread and peanut butter. Soya and mycoprotein (Quorn) are the exceptions, being 'complete' proteins in their own right.
•   The best nut varieties, protein-wise, include almonds, peanuts and pistachios. Many seeds, including hemp, pumpkin and sunflower, are also high in protein.

- Vegetables and fruit fare less well when it comes to protein content, so don't rely on them – peas (strictly a legume, rather than a vegetable) top the charts with 5.5g per 100g (3½oz) portion, broccoli has 4–5g per 100g (3½oz) (approx. half a head), a whole avocado provides 4g per 100g (3½oz) and blackberries contain 2.5g per 150g (5oz) serving (roughly one cupful).

## Making a meal of it

Including a carbohydrate-rich food and a protein-rich food at every meal is the best way to ensure you meet the requirements on a daily basis. For example, boiled egg and soldiers, baked beans on toast, tofu or chicken and rice. Then fill your plate with vegetables, salad or fruit (as a rule, vegetables and salad are mineral-rich, fruits are high in vitamins), aiming for a range of colours and types to get the greatest variety of phytonutrients.

You'll notice I haven't mentioned the other macronutrient – fat – in terms of marathon nutrition. That's not to say fat isn't an essential nutrient (important vitamins A, D, E and K are all fat soluble) – but you'll almost certainly be getting enough from the sort of diet I'm recommending (a minimum of 20 per cent of your calorie intake should derive from fat sources – the American College of Sports Medicine recommends a range between 20–35 per cent, though this is not specifically for runners). The focus should be on healthier sources of fat: omega-3 oils (oily fish, linseed, walnuts) and monounsaturated fats such as olive oil, nuts and seeds, and avocado – plus dairy, lean meats and fish, if you consume them, rather than fatty meat products, pastry, fried and processed foods, desserts and cakes.

Spreading out the macronutrients across meals ensures you are getting an overall balanced diet. But it doesn't mean you have to eat the exact same amount of each macronutrient each day. Increasingly, sports nutritionists are moving towards a more training-specific dietary prescription – with higher energy and carbohydrate intake on hard-training days and lower intakes on easy and rest days, as well as increased protein intake following hard training, to promote recovery. You can achieve this by fine-tuning your meals and snacks according to what training you will be doing, which brings us to that other major difference in the marathoner's diet – nutrient timing.

# What to eat when

Slight shifts to what and when you eat different nutrients can really make a difference to how successfully you fuel workouts and recovery.

When you are looking to fuel up for a run, carbohydrate is the nutrient to focus on. Ensuring you start your runs with enough glycogen minimises the risk of running out of energy and hitting the wall. If you run first thing and prefer not to eat beforehand, make sure you have had plenty of carbohydrate in your meal the evening before and, depending on the type of session you're doing, consider taking energy on board during the run in the form of a drink or gel (*see* 'Fuelling on the run' on p. 233).

Similarly, if you are running after work and haven't eaten since lunchtime, you may choose to boost your energy reserves pre-run with a carb-rich snack. For example, dried fruit, oatcakes, a bagel or a banana. What if you don't want to up your calorie intake through snacking? Sports dietitian Dr Karen Reid introduced me to the wonders of the 'split lunch' some years ago, and it works a treat: you simply split your lunch into two helpings, eating one at lunchtime and saving the other for mid-afternoon, thereby reducing the length of time between eating and running.

## Eating (and drinking) for recovery

After a run, the onus shifts to repair and recovery, which is when protein takes the spotlight. That's not to say that carbohydrate isn't also important at this point; stores need to be replenished – especially after long or hard runs, or when you'll be running again within the next 24 hours.

You may have heard that there is an important 'window of opportunity' for refuelling post-run, to kick-start your recovery. During this period – which extends for 30–120 minutes – your body's receptors are primed to maximise muscle glycogen storage and muscle protein synthesis, making it the perfect opportunity to refuel after a long or high-intensity run.

Before we look at what to refuel with, it's worth stressing that it is not necessary to utilise this window after every single run. If, for example, the run you completed was fairly short or easy-paced, no special recovery strategy is needed. Just wait until your next mealtime. But if you have done a fatiguing hard workout, such as interval training, or a long run, the ideal recovery prescription consists of around 1g of carbohydrate/ kg of your bodyweight (1g/2.2lb) along with 0.25–0.3g protein/kg of your bodyweight (0.25–0.3g/2.2lb). (If you don't want to worry about sums, 60g/2oz carbohydrate and 20g/⅔oz protein is a decent aim.) *See* 'Five great recovery snacks' below for some ideas.

## FIVE GREAT RECOVERY SNACKS

These snacks provide around 50–60g (1¾–2oz) of carbohydrate and 20g (⅔oz) of protein:

1. Small tin of baked beans on two slices of wholemeal toast.
2. 400ml (13½fl oz) smoothie made with semi-skimmed milk and 1 ripe banana (a pinch of cinnamon goes well). Boost the carbs with honey, if you like.
3. An apple, a pot of natural yoghurt and a palmful of mixed nuts, dried fruit and seeds.
4. A bagel with two hard-boiled eggs plus an orange.
5. 300ml (10fl oz) glass of chocolate milkshake made with soya milk and a slice of malt loaf topped with peanut butter or cottage cheese.

### Be prepared

Given that timing is everything, a little preparation might be needed to ensure that you can lay your hands on what you need when you return, ravenous, from your run or race. If finding your meal or snack of choice means waiting until you've driven the 30 miles home from a race, it'd be best to take something with you, or make do with what is available at the event. Also consider what you are able to stomach after two-plus hours of hard running. It could be that the idea of a full meal turns your stomach but you're OK with downing a chocolate milk drink or a banana smoothie. The thought of scrambled eggs on toast is what keeps me going over the last few miles of a long run!

I mentioned above that your body processes protein most efficiently when it is delivered in small, regular doses. That means you'll still need to consume protein at your next meal, even after a recovery snack. After particularly tough/long runs or races, a further protein hit before bed has been found to be beneficial in promoting muscle protein synthesis overnight. A drink or snack containing around 20g (⅔oz) of protein is usually adequate, but studies suggest that if you are aged 50 or over, a higher dose – up to 40g (1⅓oz) – is needed to get the same benefit. Milk-based options are best, because they are high in casein, which is absorbed slowly overnight.

Just to be clear, these post-workout protein recommendations are not *in addition* to the amount you've worked out you need per kg of your bodyweight per day – we're talking about how best to divide that amount up to distribute intake optimally through the day. It's better to moderate the protein portions in your main meals to allow for post-training and pre-sleep protein intake and achieve the 'small doses' approach.

After long runs, or runs on hot days, a salty food, such as pretzels or rice cakes, helps to restore electrolyte balance as well as stimulating thirst, which is handy since rehydrating is at least as important as refuelling. If you find yourself craving salty foods during your marathon training, it's worth experimenting with electrolyte drinks prior to or during running – you may be a 'salty sweater' (I'll talk more about this in the next chapter.)

## Quality vs quantity

A provocative study back in 2015 compared how well runners recovered post-exercise when they consumed proprietary 'sports nutrition' products versus fast food, in the form of a burger and chips. The researchers found that there were no differences in terms of glycogen replenishment and protein synthesis between them. However, great efforts were made to ensure that the fast-food meal supplied exactly the same nutrient quantities as the sports recovery supplement. What's more, the experiment didn't take into account the wider effects of nutrition on health. For example, a juicy burger might meet your protein requirement, but a salmon fillet would do the same, while also being rich in anti-inflammatory omega-3s. It does go to show, though, that you don't need to rely on shop-bought recovery products to get the nutrition you need – and that all foods can have a place in a runner's diet.

# Fuelling on the run

So much for tweaking your daily diet to best support marathon training. What about fuelling *during* the runs themselves? If you've read around this subject before, you could be forgiven for thinking that you should never leave the house without some carbohydrate on your person. This isn't the case.

One of the goals of marathon training is to become more proficient at burning fat as a fuel source, because it conserves or 'spares' those finite stores of muscle glycogen. Fat oxidation can increase by as much as 25 per cent through endurance training. Drip-feeding yourself with carbohydrates on every run denies your body the opportunity to become more adept at fat burning. It can also increase calorie intake unnecessarily and lower the quality of your diet, because unlike wholegrains and other healthy carbs, energy gels, sweets and drinks are a poor source of nutrients.

There are two key questions to ask yourself in determining whether to consume carbs on your run: 1) how long are you running for and 2) at what intensity?

Sport science research has clearly shown that performance in long-duration endurance exercise is improved by taking carbs on board at regular intervals to bolster dwindling glycogen stores. One study review reported improvement gains ranging from 1–13 per cent in workouts lasting 70 minutes to four hours.

The effects are most compelling when exercise lasts two to two-and-a-half hours or longer – not surprising when you consider that the muscles can only store around 400g (14oz) – 1600 calories' worth – of carbohydrate. In marathon-training for runs lasting more than two hours, I consume carbohydrate regardless of whether it's an easy run or something more pace-specific.

## Carbing up your grey matter

Studies suggest that carbohydrates can also be beneficial on shorter runs (under an hour). At first glance, this seems surprising, because muscle glycogen depletion is highly unlikely to be an issue. But researchers believe that there is another pathway through which carbohydrates can boost performance – the brain.

This was initially demonstrated in a fascinating study in which runners swished their mouths with a carbohydrate drink before spitting it out. Despite not actually swallowing the sugary liquid, they still gained performance benefits. The theory is that receptors on the tongue detect glucose (whether it is swallowed or not), which activates an area of the brain associated with reward, lowering rate of perceived exertion, dampening feelings of discomfort and boosting performance in high-intensity workouts or races. I've done this instinctively for years – taking a gel or sports drink before 10K, and 5K, races. I thought I was making doubly sure my glycogen stores were topped up, but it would appear the benefits were more cerebral!

Note, however, that this strategy is only worth employing for hard efforts, such as high-intensity workouts or races, where that reduction in perceived discomfort will be helpful. On comfortable-paced shorter runs, it's best to go carb-free.

## Going low - the pros and cons of low-carb running

Some runners choose to do a significant proportion of their runs without carbs. The aim is twofold: 1) to become more efficient at burning fat as a fuel source and 2) to supercharge the benefits they'll get when they finally do take in carbs on race day. It's a bit like not wearing your coat in the house so you 'feel the benefit' when you go outside...

This strategy, dubbed 'train low, race high', has gained purchase in the last few years. There is some solid theory behind it – studies show that when people change their diet, reducing dietary carbohydrate intake and replacing it with a higher fat intake (low carb, high fat or 'LCHF'), fat oxidation (burning) increases. However, this doesn't necessarily translate into a performance gain: one study in which race walkers adopted a LCHF diet found that despite greater fat oxidation, their economy went down and they experienced a performance *decline*. In addition, carb-depleted training increases perceived effort, which makes it unlikely that you'll be able to achieve (or maintain) the same level of intensity in training, thereby limiting your opportunity for training adaptations.

Another potential drawback is that by shunning carbs in training, you don't become accustomed to the habit of taking them in 'on the run', both in terms of gut comfort and dexterity in opening gels or chewing sweets. Come race day, you may suddenly find out that your body isn't happy chowing down carbs! And, as mentioned above, a low-carbohydrate diet appears to have a negative effect on the immune system.

The area within running where a LCHF diet does seem to make more sense is ultrarunning, where distance, rather than pace, is the main focus. Anecdotally, many ultrarunners say that they have performed better after switching to this way of eating.

If you are intrigued and want to give it a go, proceed with caution. Rather than setting out on your 18 mile (30km)-long run with no carbs to hand, try going carb-free on moderate-length runs and on the occasional hard workout or race (such as a 10K or 10-miler/16km) first and see how your body responds. Eliminating carbs from your pre-run meal is another way of limiting your glycogen supply.

## Carb intake guidelines

Sports nutritionists recommend an intake of 30–60g (1–2oz) carbs per hour during endurance exercise.

Higher intakes – 70–90g (2½–3oz) carbohydrate per hour – are sometimes recommended for exercise lasting more than two-and-a-half hours, but the risk of gastrointestinal distress is higher and these rates are only really relevant for people who are not just exercising for a long duration but doing so at a high percentage of their maximum capacity, such as someone running under three hours for the marathon.

To get a discernible benefit in runs or races where depletion of glycogen is a genuine prospect (which covers pretty much every runner's marathon), 30g (1oz) of carbohydrate per hour really is a minimum target. And yet Spanish research in 2020 found that runners participating in a 18.6-mile (30km) race took in on average just under 15g (½oz) per hour.

I suspect this is partly because many people don't have a clear idea of what 30g (1oz) or 60g (2oz) of carbohydrate actually looks like, in terms of a sports nutrition product. I had a delve in my cupboard and here's what I've found:

- 1 bottle of Lucozade sport contains 31g, so 30–60g (1–2oz) is the equivalent of drinking one or two bottles (per hour, in all cases).
- 1 Torq energy gel contains 28g, so 30–60g is the equivalent of one or two energy gels.
- 1 Jelly Baby contains 5.25g carbs, so 30–60g is the equivalent of 6–12 Jelly Babies.
- 1 Clif Blok energy chew contains 7.5g so 30–60g is the equivalent of four to eight sweets.

Different brands vary, both in size of container and content, so look at the labels of your preferred products.

What about real food? Some people struggle with – or simply don't like – the commercial options available and prefer to stick to 'real' food. The challenge is to find something that is portable, easy to eat on the move and that will deliver a good amount of carbohydrate and little else (since fat and fibre will hamper swift absorption). Use nutrition labels to figure out how much carbohydrate your chosen food will provide. Good options include a ripe banana, pitted dates or a handful of pretzels.

## Start early and fuel regularly

Whatever your choice, don't wait until you feel like you *need* an energy boost to start consuming carbs on the run. You should begin within the first half hour of running and top up at regular intervals thereafter. My personal plan for a marathon is to take an energy gel just before the start and another every 40–45 minutes. I'll take water from the aid stations and if the sports drink they are offering is a brand I'm familiar with, or if I come across someone offering Jelly Babies, I'll take these too, for a change of texture and taste. In the next chapter, I'll explain why I rely more on gels than sports drinks for my carbohydrates.

I know a lot of people have misgivings about energy gels – branding them all sticky and sickly. I'd argue that there are so many options out there, it's definitely possible to find a consistency and flavour that works for you. Some are quite runny, others you could almost chew! It's worth trying a few brands and flavours before you dismiss all gels just because of one revolting experience. Another common criticism is that you 'need to take them with water'. This is true, but it's not because they require diluting, it's because there isn't sufficient fluid within a pocket-sized sachet to keep you hydrated.

If you have struggled in the past with consuming carbs on the run, do try to persevere. To make things easier for yourself, consume your chosen source in two or three 'doses' over a few minutes rather than all at once. The gastrointestinal system does adapt, and over time you'll be able to handle it better and will benefit from doing so.

I would go so far as to say that taking on additional carbohydrate energy in marathon training and racing is vital, if you want to perform to your maximum potential. Now is the time to start to experiment with one or all of the options outlined here – even if thus far you've never taken energy on board during a run or have already run marathons before without doing so.

Before we leave the topic of carbohydrate and glycogen stores behind, I want to share with you a fascinating fact. Muscle glycogen doesn't *literally* run out. Studies show that even when an endurance athlete reaches exhaustion, there is still some glycogen present in the muscle tissues. So why can't they keep going? The brain has made it unavailable – so as far as your exercising muscles are concerned, the well is dry. Sport scientists believe this is a protective mechanism and you can read more about how the brain influences the body's performance in Chapter 6.

# 18

# GOOD HYDRATION

## What and when to drink

Most runners are now familiar with the advice to 'drink to thirst' during running, rather than attempting to drink a specific amount at set intervals.

This reflects two important facts: one, that there are big differences in the amount that individuals sweat – a combination of genetics and body size (bigger people sweat more). Two, that many factors influence sweat rate – how intensely you are exercising (you'll sweat more if you are running at 5K pace than if you are just jogging), what you are wearing, the conditions/temperature you are running in (humidity has a big impact on sweat's ability to evaporate from skin) and how accustomed you are to running in those particular conditions (you acclimatise).

Fitness level is another factor. Research from Korea found that runners break into a sweat more quickly than sedentary people – suggesting that with training and improved fitness, the body becomes more efficient at regulating heat. There's also the matter of your personal tolerance for drinking – or not drinking – during exercise. I'm a guzzler, while my husband is a lizard!

All of the above makes it impossible – or at least unwise – to give a specific volume recommendation of how much to drink on the run. Research has shown that sweat rates per hour of running can range from 0.4–1.8 litres (0.7–3 pints). If two runners, one at each end of this range, were given a specific volume of fluid per hour to drink, one would likely not replace *enough* lost fluids, while the other would be drinking far in excess of what they'd lost. Better for each to drink when they feel like it.

This is borne out by a study, published in the journal *Sports Medicine*, which compared endurance performance when people drank a prescribed amount with performance when they drank *ad libitum* (with free choice). Those on the prescribed amount consumed twice as much fluid as those drinking when they felt like it and became less dehydrated (as measured by a change in bodyweight) but – and it's a big but! – performance did *not* improve as a result. In fact, the *ad libitum* exercisers performed a bit better.

## Advice for non-drinkers

So far, so good. Drink to thirst. But what if you're one of those people who is *never* thirsty during runs? Forcing down fluid isn't 'drinking to thirst' is it? Well, no. And for runs of an hour or less, I wouldn't worry about it. But when it comes to training runs of 90 minutes or more, I'd recommend trying to get accustomed to taking on some fluid – because the longer the extent of a run, the greater the amount of water you lose through sweat and the higher the risk of this impacting on your performance (especially if it's hot or humid, or you're running at pace – or all three).

Let's take a 70kg (11 stone) runner with an average sweat rate of 1 litre (1.75 pints) per hour (I've picked the middle of the 0.4–1.8 litre/0.7–3 pints range outlined above) who doesn't customarily drink on the run. During a two-hour half-marathon, our runner will lose 2 litres (3.5 pints) of sweat, which is equivalent to 2.8 per cent of their bodyweight – a level of dehydration that isn't too concerning (despite the oft-quoted contention that even 2 per cent dehydration will have a detrimental impact on performance). But if that 70kg runner goes on to run a marathon in four-and-a-half hours with no fluid, they stand to lose 4.5 litres (7.9 pints) of sweat, equivalent to a much more concerning (in terms of health and performance) 6.4 per cent of their bodyweight. If I were coaching this person, I'd recommend that they try scheduling a drink every 3 miles (5km) or every 30 minutes, rather than relying on their (non-existent!) thirst. As with carbohydrate intake, you can 'train' yourself to drink during running, even if you currently find it difficult to tolerate. (*See* 'Five drinking tips for runners' on p. 243.)

Another important point to bear in mind is that hydration isn't just about what you do during that hour – or three – when you are running.

One study found that beginning exercise in a hypo-hydrated (slightly dehydrated) state decreased endurance exercise performance by 2.4 per cent compared to a well-hydrated state. If you make the effort to stay well hydrated during your daily life by drinking to thirst (even if that means asking yourself regularly 'am I thirsty?') you are less likely to *start* runs in a dehydrated state, which takes the pressure of needing to drink during the run simply to get back on an even keel.

Checking your urine colour is a useful indicator of your hydration status – dark-coloured urine suggests you're not drinking enough. Also consider pee frequency and volume.

## What are electrolytes – and do I need them?

It's not just water that is lost in sweat. The body also loses electrolytes – mineral salts – in the form of sodium, potassium and chloride. Just as we all sweat vastly different amounts, we also lose different amounts of electrolytes (particularly sodium) in our sweat. Precision Hydration, specialists in sports hydration assessment, report that they've seen levels vary from 200mg/litre (200mg/1.75 pints) to 2300mg/litre (2300mg/1.75 pints)! If you're a salty sweater – someone who has high concentrations of sodium in their sweat – you may well have noticed white 'tide marks' on your T-shirt when running on a hot day or noticed that your sweat tastes particularly salty, or stings your eyes.

Sports drinks – along with most gels – contain electrolytes to help you replace what you lose through sweat. But because individual losses are so different, the amount supplied in a drink (typically 250–300mg of sodium) may not meet your needs. That's where electrolyte drinks or tablets (that you pop into water or a sports drink) come in. Precision Hydration offer a free hydration plan, based on your responses to a questionnaire, on their website (*see* Resources). I often add an electrolyte tablet to the bottle of water that I drink in the 24 hours leading up to an important long run or race, to help mitigate losses.

## Dehydration and hyponatraemia

A 2012 study estimated the average level of dehydration among marathon race winners at the finish line was 8.8 per cent – far in excess of the 2 per cent that is often said to be the level at which performance will be negatively impacted. I'm not mentioning this to imply that dehydration doesn't present a risk – higher heart rate and blood pressure (due to 'thicker' blood that takes more work to pump around the body), increased rate of perceived exertion and elevated levels of cortisol, the 'stress' hormone, are all unwelcome consequences of underhydration. You may also get muscle cramps or headaches, or feel dizzy and confused.

However, minor levels of dehydration are not dangerous, or even necessarily detrimental to performance. In fact, back in 1968, the winner of the Boston Marathon, Amby Burfoot, didn't drink any fluid at all. I don't recommend following in his footsteps, but I wouldn't get overly concerned about becoming dehydrated as long as you have access to a drink and abide by your thirst. This should hold true even on hot and humid days, when fluid needs are greater, because your 'thirst drive' will be higher.

But use your common sense. If your mouth feels dry, have a drink. If your stomach is sloshing around with fluid, don't. What colour is your pee? Do you keep having to stop to duck into the bushes or find a race Portaloo? What's the weather like? How are you feeling? How long have you been running for?

At the opposite end of the hydration spectrum from dehydration lies exercise-associated hyponatraemia (EAH). EAH is a condition in which excessive fluid intake – combined with loss of sodium through sweat – dilutes the body's sodium levels to an extent that it cannot perform normal regulatory processes.

Unfortunately, some of the symptoms of EAH are the same as those of dehydration, making it all the more important to be mindful about how much you are drinking. Serious and fatal cases of EAH mostly occur when people have drunk too much water over a prolonged period of exertion. This is why it's more common among marathon runners – who have ample access to fluid during the hours they are racing – than in, say, footballers or tennis players, for whom the opportunities to drink are far fewer. Studies have showed that those most at risk tend to be runners who are out on the course for longer than four hours, who drink at every aid station and end up consuming in excess of 3 litres (5.3 pints) by the finish. If this sounds like it might apply to you, it's worth factoring electrolytes into your hydration plan, or alternating between water and sports drink.

The bottom line? Don't worry too much about falling prey to either dehydration or hyponatraemia: if you drink to thirst and with awareness, use your common sense and seek assistance if you feel unwell during or after the race, you should be fine.

## FIVE DRINKING TIPS FOR RUNNERS

- Stop drinking an hour before the race start, and visit the loo.
- Just before the gun goes, drink some fluid. As blood diverts away from the digestive system to the exercising muscles, this will not 'go straight through you'.
- As a vague guideline, six to eight gulps of fluid are equivalent to around 200ml (6.8fl oz).
- Take the drink into your mouth with your throat closed. Then close your mouth and open your throat to swallow it. If you try to guzzle it straight down while you are moving up and down from the running action, you are more likely to risk a choking fit.
- Room-temperature fluid is generally easier on your guts than icy cold.

## What to drink

Water is my fluid of choice on the run, because I like to separate my carbohydrate and fluid needs. That way, I can take as much carbohydrate as I need (in the form of gels or sweets) irrespective of how thirsty I am.

The other option is to drink sports drink. Look out for the term 'isotonic' on the label – many so-called energy drinks are *not* isotonic. This term refers to the concentration of dissolved particles (sugars and salts) in a fluid. When a fluid is isotonic, its concentration is the same as the fluid in the body's cells – and the important thing about this is that it means it will be transported from the gut to the bloodstream more quickly to deliver its 'wares' (hydration, energy, electrolytes). If a drink is isotonic, its carbohydrate content will be 6–8 per cent – any higher than that and the absorption rate will be slower.

When it comes to really long runs, opting for sports drinks presents a potential problem. Why? Well, one 500ml (17fl oz) bottle of sports drink contains roughly the same amount of carbs as an energy gel – 25–30g (c. 1oz). To get 30–60g (1–2oz) carbohydrate, you would need to drink one or two bottles of sports drink per hour. In a four-hour marathon, that could mean four to eight bottles' worth. Such a high volume of liquid could feel like too much, leaving your stomach feeling uncomfortable. Energy gels eliminate this risk. One compromise is to alternate between sports drink and energy gels/sweets to ensure you get your 30–60g carbohydrate per hour. It's a myth that you can't 'mix' the two – but I would recommend drinking the sports drink on its own and taking the gels/sweets with a little water, rather than washing them down with sports drink.

## Putting it all into practice

It's really important that you use your long training runs to experiment with different fuel and hydration strategies. And once you've nailed it, practise, practise, practise! This is what gets your body accustomed to absorbing carbohydrate and fluid while on the move without being hampered by gastrointestinal complaints. You can read more about fuelling up specifically for race day in Chapter 15.

# 19

# ERGOGENIC AIDS AND ESSENTIAL NUTRIENTS

## Read if you want to go faster...

When something is described as 'ergogenic', it means that it enhances physical performance. By that definition, carbohydrate – or even water – could be considered ergogenic; but the term is most commonly used to describe nutritional supplements and substances taken solely for a performance boost. In researching this chapter, I came across claims for everything from omega-3 fatty acids to ginseng, sodium phosphate to beta-alanine. The scientific research on the majority of these is unconvincing, equivocal or in the early stages and too soon to draw conclusions from, so I've limited inclusion to the two substances that have widespread and convincing evidence specifically in relation to endurance activities like marathon running.

## Caffeine

After hydration and energy provision, the single best bet for a performance boost is caffeine. It's the most widely studied ergogenic aid and, happily for us runners, a 2021 review from the International Society of Sports Nutrition shows that it works its magic most reliably and consistently in aerobic endurance exercise.

The review collated the findings of dozens of studies and reported a small but significant 2–4 per cent average improvement in endurance performance when taken in doses equal to 3–6mg/kg (3–6mg/2.2lb) body mass. (For a 70kg/11 stone runner, that's 210–420mg. As a point of comparison, a Costa Coffee flat white contains 277mg of caffeine.) Individual studies have found far greater improvements – one noted an average performance improvement of 11.2 per cent with caffeine use.

The ergogenic effect of caffeine relates mostly to the central nervous system, with studies showing a reduction in perceived effort during exercise (the study mentioned above found a 5.6 per cent reduction in RPE), less muscle pain and a greater capacity to exert muscular force. Improvements in attention and concentration during exercise – and even energy and mood – have also been reported.

Caffeine is rapidly absorbed from the stomach and intestines. It appears in the blood within minutes of ingestion, but its peak concentration comes 30–120 minutes later. That's why it is most often recommended as a pre-exercise hit. However, some recent studies have found that it also serves well in providing a boost late on during prolonged endurance exercise. For example, a cycling study found that when caffeine was consumed 80 minutes into a 120-minute time trial, it significantly improved performance compared to when a placebo was taken. Both a low dose (1.5mg/kg or 1.5mg/2.2lb of bodyweight) and a higher dose (3mg/kg or 3mg/2.2lb of bodyweight) had an effect, though the higher dose made a greater difference.

As far as marathon training is concerned, the key message is to consider adding mid-race caffeine to your nutrition plan, rather than just a single pre-exercise dose. Which brings us to the question, how should I take my caffeine?

A pre-training or racing fix may come in the form of good old coffee. (Research comparing the performance effects of caffeine consumed in its pure form or in coffee found no significant difference – but the 'dose' delivered in each case was identical, which is less easy to achieve outside of a laboratory setting.) But assuming you're not going to be stopping for a double espresso at mile 18, you'll need to look elsewhere for a mid-race pick-me-up, and happily, there is an increasing choice of proprietary caffeinated products for athletes, including gels, drinks, shots, sweets, chewing gum (particularly quickly absorbed and the least demanding on the digestive system) and even oral sprays.

As mentioned, doses equal to 3–6mg/kg (3–6mg/2.2lb) of bodyweight are the most widely tried and tested. But lower doses have also been found to be effective. Remember, studies report what the 'average' response was – some people will experience a more profound effect than average and some, no effect at all.

## Individual differences

The most likely factor influencing the extent of an individual's response to caffeine is genetic variation. Some people's gene expression renders them 'high responsive' while others are 'low responsive' or even 'non-responsive'. In fact, some studies have found individuals whose performance *worsens* with caffeine. You will need to experiment and see what works for you – and indeed, *if* it works for you. A cautious starting point would be a single dose of around 100mg.

If you are a coffee addict, you may wonder whether your caffeine habit numbs the ergogenic effect. The most up-to-date research suggests that the benefits endure even in regular caffeine users.

Researchers have also looked at the question of whether to get the greatest benefit from caffeine for performance, you should abstain from it in the days leading up to your event. Personally, I'd be worried that any potential benefit would be negated by the splitting headache I always get when I forgo my morning coffee, so I was glad to find a high-quality double-blinded, placebo-controlled study that noted equal beneficial effects on time trial performance, regardless of whether people abstained from caffeine for four days beforehand or not. Phew!

## Dietary nitrates (beetroot juice)

Another diet-derived substance you may have come across if you've ever looked into performance-enhancing aids for runners is beetroot juice. Since the mid-2000s, numerous studies have been published showing that beetroot juice – due to its high concentration of dietary nitrates – can improve endurance, whether that is measured by time to exhaustion or time to complete a specific distance. This appears to be due to enhanced oxygen delivery to the working muscles, and improved mitochondrial efficiency. Beetroot juice has also been found to improve 'exercise tolerance' in moderately trained people – enabling them to work harder without feeling as if they are.

In a review of more than 80 studies on the effects of beetroot on exercise performance in October 2020, researchers concluded that while findings were mixed, there was a clear, though small, ergogenic effect. It seems like a no-brainer to stain your lips (and your wee) pink, then. But the truth is a little more complex. Many factors seem to impact how ergogenic dietary nitrate is.

The clearest one is fitness level. The evidence definitely points towards there being significantly less benefit among those who are highly trained and extremely fit compared to us lesser mortals! This is different to caffeine, where the magnitude of performance improvement has not been found to differ between recreational and elite athletes. The review mentioned above raises the issue of gender differences – reporting that women-only studies have found a more blunted response to dietary nitrate compared to mixed studies or those only on men. But they also point out that women are underrepresented in the research, so it could be that further studies refute this.

## What's the dose?

There is also the matter of how much to consume, how often and in what form. The recommended 'dose' is 5–25mmol (a millimole is a measurement of a chemical substance) of dietary nitrate, with many studies issuing subjects with one or two commercial beetroot juice 'shots', containing around 6.5mmol each. Timing is everything. Leaving less than 90 minutes between consumption and exercise resulted in no benefit, while consuming two to three-and-a-half hours beforehand produced the best results. Interestingly, the study review did not find any differences between taking a single dose and 'pre-loading' over several days (a common practice among beetroot juice aficionados).

Can you get enough dietary nitrate from drinking normal beetroot juice, instead of proprietary shots? You can; but while a shot is around 70ml (2.4fl oz), you'd need to drink 500ml (16.9fl oz) of juice to get the equivalent nitrate from normal beet juice. Of course, beetroot isn't the only source. Other fruit and veg that are high in nitrates include rhubarb, celery, rocket, lettuce and spinach.

The bottom line? Given that some studies have found no response, others a response from a single dose and others only from a repeated dose, it's a matter of trying it out for yourself. As with caffeine, there are likely to be people who are highly responsive and those who are non-responsive.

## Nutrients to watch

The nutrients included in the following section are not ergogenic aids, in the sense that they won't enhance your performance simply by taking them. However, in the case of the vitamins and minerals, a deficiency can certainly harm performance and/or raise injury risk, while probiotics can play an important role in supporting the immune system and reducing the risk of gastrointestinal problems in running.

### Calcium

Calcium is well known for its role in bone health – which makes it a crucial nutrient for anyone who is stressing their bones through the impact of running. In addition, calcium plays an important role in muscular contraction, nerve function and heart rhythm. Women in particular should take care to consume enough calcium (the UK RDA is 700mg) because of the acceleration of bone loss post-menopause, leading to an increased risk of osteoporosis.

Recent research suggests that calcium consumed prior to exercise (an hour or two beforehand) can diminish the usual exercise-induced increase in parathyroid hormone (a hormone that causes the release of calcium from bone), which helps protect against bone mineral loss. This benefit has been found in studies using calcium-rich meals as well as using supplementation of 1g of calcium (1000mg).

Dairy products are the best source of calcium – the 'bioavailability' of the calcium in milk and milk-derived foods is higher than it is in many plant-based foods – but other good sources include soya beans, tofu, chickpeas, canned sardines (which contain the bones), fortified cereals, almonds and broccoli. Vegans are advised to replace milk and dairy with calcium-enriched soya products or other fortified plant-based milks.

# Vitamin D

Like calcium, vitamin D is important in maintaining good bone health. The relationship between vitamin D status and injury prevention (including a decreased risk of stress fracture) and rehabilitation has been well documented.

But with the discovery of vitamin D receptors in muscle and immune system cells, scientific interest has increased and widened. A growing number of studies have found links between vitamin D status and neuromuscular function, muscle fibre size, levels of inflammation and immune response (particularly to respiratory illness).

Yet research suggests that many of us are not getting enough vitamin D, particularly in the winter months, when there isn't sufficient sunlight to stimulate the body into making its own vitamin D. A 2017 study found the prevalence of vitamin D deficiency in the UK was approximately 24 per cent in men and 21 per cent in women aged between 19 and 64.

Good dietary sources of vitamin D are few and far between – oily fish, eggs and fortified products – which is why Public Health England recommends people take 10ug/micrograms, the equivalent of 400iu/international units, of vitamin D between October and March. (Make sure your supplement is vitamin D3, which has better bioavailability than D2).

However, many studies within an athletics context use significantly greater amounts than this – for example, one study in 2020 used a daily dose of 6000iu for six weeks to correct a deficiency, resulting in improved performance.

This raises an important point: how much vitamin D you consume isn't as important as what level you end up with in your blood. That's why scientific studies typically measure blood serum levels of vitamin D and monitor changes to it in response to supplementation.

In the UK, a blood serum level of below 25nmol/L is considered to mark a vitamin D deficiency. This is a lower benchmark than many other countries. In the United States, a level below 30nmol/L is considered deficient, with readings between 30 and 49nmol/L considered 'inadequate'. In Australia, anything below 50nmol/L is considered deficient.

The best way to find out if you might benefit from supplementation in excess of the nationally recommended winter dose of 400iu is to have your vitamin D levels tested. This can be done by your GP (though in the absence of ill health, they may not agree to it) or with a home-testing kit.

What level should you be looking to achieve? Well, a 2021 review of vitamin D sufficiency in athletes recommends aiming for blood serum levels of 80–100nmol/L. This ties in with a 2016 study that recommended athletes in hard training aim to maintain a reading of 75nmol/L. Certainly, if your level is below 50nmol/L, you would be advised to up your daily dose.

## Iron

Iron is involved in the formation of red blood cells and the transportation of oxygen to all the body's cells, making it a precious metal to any runner. A low iron status can hamper athletic performance by impairing muscle function and limiting work capacity as well as lessening adaptation to endurance training.

Iron deficiency is not uncommon in the Western world as a whole and a 2019 study estimates as many as 15–35 per cent of female athletes could have an iron deficiency. Intense training can increase losses of the mineral through sweat, urination and the gastrointestinal tract. There's also something called 'foot strike haemolysis', in which (so the theory goes) red blood cells are compressed and damaged in the feet.

Do runners need more iron then? The consensus is no. But it is very important that you meet the recommended daily intake guidelines – 14.8mg of iron per day for women (pre menopause) and 8.7mg per day for men and post-menopausal women. Runners who are most at risk of deficiency are women (due to menstruation, so especially true of those with heavy periods), people on low-calorie diets (who are more at risk of deficiencies of any type), vegetarians and vegans. The latter two are susceptible because 'haem' iron from animal sources is better absorbed than 'non-haem' plant-derived sources. But rather than taking a supplement 'just to be safe', it's best to have your iron levels assessed and only take it if you need it. Iron supplements can be stressful on the stomach and excessive doses can be toxic.

We tend to think of iron-deficiency as anaemia, but there is also a condition called iron deficiency non anaemia (IDNA), where haemoglobin levels are normal but ferritin levels (how the body stores iron) are low. If you suspect you might be iron deficient (symptoms include fatigue, shortness of breath, sub-par performances and 'heavy' legs) the best thing to do is to get both haemoglobin and ferritin levels tested.

## Make the most of your iron intake...

☑ Choose haem sources if you can, such as red meat (especially liver) and eggs. Good non-haem sources include beans and pulses, iron-fortified breakfast cereals and dark green vegetables such as spinach and kale.

☑ Avoid tea with iron-rich foods or supplements – the tannins it contains hamper absorption.

☑ Eat or drink something rich in vitamin C with your iron source. Studies show that this can increase absorption threefold.

☑ Don't take calcium and iron supplements at the same time. Leave several hours between them.

## Probiotics

The importance of maintaining a healthy gut or 'microbiome' has come to the fore over the last few years. The gut naturally contains trillions of bacteria that help keep us healthy. They play a big role in immune function, help prevent gastrointestinal disturbances (such as stomach bugs, diarrhoea and constipation) and may even influence mood and mental health. With a nutritious, minimally processed diet and healthy lifestyle, the gut should take care of itself. But when the body is under more stress than usual, through prolonged periods of hard training, for example, or a less-than-ideal diet, it may benefit from some support, in the form of 'good' (friendly) bacteria present in food products such as live yoghurt or fermented foods like sauerkraut, kefir or kimchi, or in supplement form.

In one study, published in the *British Journal of Sports Medicine*, 20 elite distance runners who supplemented with probiotics during four months of winter training experienced milder symptoms and shorter bouts of respiratory illness. Other research has found that supplementation can reduce GI issues in runners by helping to restore the lining of the gut. Probiotics may also help to increase the uptake of iron – particularly important for female runners, who are more likely to suffer from iron deficiency.

I don't take probiotics routinely, but now and again, I take a course of them either because I feel my body is under a lot of stress or because my guts aren't playing nicely. Another time when they can be particularly helpful is following a course of antibiotics, which will wipe out not just the 'unfriendly' bacteria in your gut but the good guys, too.

# CONCLUSION

When I set out to write this book, my aim was to offer runners more than a series of 'how to' instructions on marathon running, with a choice of off-the-shelf training programmes.

The formula for creating a successful training plan is Athlete + Goal = Training Plan.

When you choose a finish-time-based training plan, the formula isn't complete – it's just 'Goal', without any consideration of 'Athlete'. Often, such an approach falls short.

Throughout this book, I've included up-to-date research-backed information and expert advice on every aspect of marathon training. But I have also tried to show runners how to bring themselves into the equation when deciding on the right approach to take, be it whether to add plyometrics to their training schedule or electrolytes to their drinks. Bringing yourself into the equation means factoring in everything from your age to experience level, natural ability to injury propensity, mental attitude to sweat rate. The more you know about yourself as a runner – mentally and physically – the easier it is to make the right decisions about how to hone marathon training to suit you as an individual.

You may not agree with everything in this book. You may not find everything in it works for you. As I've said, there is no single 100% effective method of preparing to run a marathon (borne out by the fact that there are many successful coaches and athletes who don't share the same approach). But whether it be related to mindset or mileage, fuel or footwear, you will be armed with the necessary information and know-how to adapt, or try alternatives to, the practices and strategies I've suggested.

It is a bold move to call this book *Run Your Best Marathon*! As all runners know, a lot of stars need to line up to make everything go perfectly on race day – including some things that are outside of our control, like the temperature or wind speed. The most we can do is turn up at the start line knowing that we have done the best we can to prepare, with a clear race plan in mind and the focus and determination to carry it out. Crossing the finish line knowing that you achieved that is something to be proud of, regardless of the time on the clock.

Running your best marathon needn't be a one-off opportunity either. For those who are taking on the distance for the first time, a PB is guaranteed, but it's likely that future efforts will improve on your debut race, thanks to all the knowledge and experience you will glean along the way. Experienced runners may find that employing a fresh approach to training achieves the breakthrough they were looking for, but even then, there will always be something more to address, tweak or improve on.

My hope is that first-timers and marathon veterans alike will find themselves returning to this book over and over in their continued quest to run and race better.

I'll leave you with the words of Eliud Kipchoge:

'With a strong heart and a good mind, you can do it.'

# REFERENCES

## Chapter 1

'... 33 per cent higher capillarisation in endurance athletes compared to non-active people'
'Capillary supply of skeletal muscle fibers in untrained and endurance-trained men', PubMed (nih.gov)

'The fastest-growing age group participating in marathons in 2014–2017 was 90–99-year-olds!'
'Marathon Statistics 2021 Worldwide Average Finishing Times' (runnerclick.com)

## Chapter 2

'... this did not translate to better performance'
'Skeletal muscle adaptation and performance responses to once a day versus twice every second day endurance training regimens', *Journal of Applied Physiology*

## Chapter 3

'Other research...suggests that women perceive the 'best' time, performance wise, is just after bleeding has ceased (the late follicular phase).'
'Changes in Self-Reported Physical Fitness, Performance, and Side Effects Across the Phases of the Menstrual Cycle Among Competitive Endurance Athletes', PubMed (nih.gov)

'...women consistently identify a drop in performance during the early follicular and late luteal phases'.

'The Impact of Menstrual Cycle Phases on Athlete's Performance: A Narrative Review', PubMed (nih.gov)

## Chapter 5

'... increased the workload of the ankle musculature by around 20 per cent compared to flat ground'
'Biomechanics and energetics of running on uneven terrain', PubMed (nih.gov)

'... the energy cost of running at a specific pace on an irregular surface was 10 per cent greater than on a level one'
'Kinematics and metabolic cost of running on an irregular treadmill surface', PubMed (nih.gov)

'... and peak propulsive force (the force applied to the ground during 'take off') lower'
'Is Motorized Treadmill Running Biomechanically Comparable to Overground Running? A Systematic Review and Meta-Analysis of Cross-Over Studies', PubMed (nih.gov)

'... faster running creates more heat, which may be dispersed less efficiently indoors)'
'A Systematic Review and Meta-Analysis of Crossover Studies Comparing Physiological, Perceptual and Performance Measures Between Treadmill and Overground Running', PubMed (nih.gov)

'... greater muscle activity, especially from those glutes'
'Biomechanics and Physiology of Uphill and Downhill Running', PubMed (nih.gov)

'... it's important to include a range of different types of hill training'
'Effects of different uphill interval-training programs on running economy and performance', PubMed (nih.gov)

'... higher loading rate (especially at the knee joint) and impact force, which could raise injury risk'
'The effects of downhill slope on kinematics and kinetics of the lower extremity joints during running', PubMed (nih.gov)
'Downhill Running: What Are The Effects and How Can We Adapt? A Narrative Review', PubMed (nih.gov) 2020
'Effect of downhill running grade on lower extremity loading in female distance runners', PubMed (nih.gov)
'... overweight people lost more weight when they exercised in the morning'
'Consistent Morning Exercise May Be Beneficial for Individuals With Obesity', PubMed (nih.gov)

'... a hormone associated with readiness to sleep'
'Influence of Exercise Time of Day on Salivary Melatonin Responses', PubMed (nih.gov)

'Time of day has been shown to impact on athletic performance, too'
'The effect of training at a specific time of day: a review', PubMed (nih.gov)

'Indeed, the evidence overall strongly suggests that athletic performance is best in the evening'
'Sleep, circadian rhythms, and athletic performance', PubMed (nih.gov)

'... more consistent (amassing more training time overall) than those who exercise at more random times'

'Relationship of Consistency in Timing of Exercise Performance and Exercise Levels Among Successful Weight Loss Maintainers', PubMed (nih.gov)

'... when the timing of the workout chimes with our chronotype'
'Chronotype, Physical Activity, and Sport Performance: A Systematic Review', PubMed (nih.gov)

'... they coped better with the morning workout due to their chronotype'
'Salivary cortisol concentration after high-intensity interval exercise: Time of day and chronotype effect', PubMed (nih.gov)

'... are more likely to be "morning" types' www.ncbi.nlm.nih.gov/pmc/articles/PMC5187972

'... this practice may enhance training adaptations and boost the immune system'
'Taking a hot bath after exercise improves performance in the heat' (theconversation.com)

## Chapter 6

'... the effects of listening to music *during* running'
'Effects of Preferred and Nonpreferred Warm-Up Music on Exercise Performance', PubMed (nih.gov)

'... not given any instructions about entrainment'
'Instructed versus spontaneous entrainment of running cadence to music tempo', PubMed (nih.gov)

'... focusing on breathing or the movement of the body actually *worsens* running economy'
'Thinking about your running movement makes you less efficient: attentional focus effects on running economy and kinematics', PubMed (nih.gov)

'... does not have a negative impact on economy'
'An internal focus of attention is not always as bad as its reputation: how specific aspects of internally focused attention do not hinder running efficiency', PubMed (nih.gov)

'... just as adding more physical training would' www.ncbi.nlm.nih.gov/pubmed/19131473 https://pubmed.ncbi.nlm.nih.gov/28044281/

'... faster in a time trial than in the same test performed alone' www.ncbi.nlm.nih.gov/pubmed/26726003

## Chapter 7

'... a landmark study in the *British Journal of Sports Medicine*'
'Running shoes and running injuries: mythbusting and a proposal for two new paradigms: "preferred movement path" and "comfort filter"', *British Journal of Sports Medicine* (bmj.com)

'... a US trial with over 7000 subjects'
http://10.0.9.215/jospt.2014.5342

'... the role of running shoe technology in injury prevention has been largely overrated'
'Can the "Appropriate" Footwear Prevent Injury in Leisure-Time Running? Evidence Versus Beliefs', *Journal of Athletic Training* (allenpress.com)

## Chapter 8

'... a small decrease in the level of post-exercise muscle soreness when a warm-up is performed'
'Warm-up reduces delayed onset muscle soreness but cool-down does not: a randomised controlled trial', PubMed (nih.gov)

'... foam rolling helps to improve joint range of motion prior to exercise'
'A Meta-Analysis of the Effects of Foam Rolling on Performance and Recovery', PubMed (nih.gov)

'... foam rolling before exercise had an additional positive effect compared to either modality alone'
'The Accumulated Effects of Foam Rolling Combined with Stretching on Range of Motion and Physical Performance: A Systematic Review and Meta-Analysis' (nih.gov)

'... rolling in each direction for two to four seconds'
'Foam Rolling Prescription: A Clinical Commentary', PubMed (nih.gov)

'... compared to low and moderate pain perception'
'Higher Quadriceps Roller Massage Forces Do Not Amplify Range-of-Motion Increases nor Impair Strength and Jump Performance', PubMed (nih.gov)

'... isn't a helpful thing to do before a run' www.ncbi.nlm.nih.gov/pmc/articles/PMC6895680/

'... stretching for shorter durations ... has a much less significant impact'

D.G. Behm, A.J. Blazevich, A.D. Kay, M. McHugh, 'Acute effects of muscle stretching on physical performance, range of motion, and injury incidence in healthy active individuals: a systematic review', *Applied Physiology, Nutrition, and Metabolism*, 2016 Jan; 41(1):1–11

'... followed up with more dynamic activity, any performance detriment is restored'
https://pubmed.ncbi.nlm.nih.gov/26642915/

'... its potential positive effect on flexibility and musculotendinous injury prevention'
www.ncbi.nlm.nih.gov/pmc/articles/PMC6895680/

'... no clear effect of static stretching on all-cause or overuse injuries'
https://pubmed.ncbi.nlm.nih.gov/18785063/

'... how quickly the "stress response" can be switched off' https://pubmed
.ncbi.nlm.nih.gov/12735426/
and ref 135 here: www.ncbi.nlm.nih.gov/pmc/articles/PMC5999142/#CR105

'... did indeed lead to a more rapid return to a resting state' https://pubmed
.ncbi.nlm.nih.gov/12735426/

'... concluded that a cool-down did not speed recovery or prevent DOMS'
www.ncbi.nlm.nih.gov/pmc/articles/PMC5999142/

'... almost two-thirds of marathon runners include post-run stretching'
'Course and predicting factors of lower-extremity injuries after running a
marathon', PubMed (nih.gov)

'... the extent to which it reduced soreness the day after exercise was
equivalent to one point on a 100-point scale'
'Stretching to prevent or reduce muscle soreness after exercise', PubMed
(nih.gov)

## Chapter 9

'... a fascinating study conducted back in 2014'

'Postexercise cold water immersion benefits are not greater than the
placebo effect', PubMed (nih.gov)

'... three times greater in the group whose muscles were *not* cooled after training'
https://pubmed.ncbi.nlm.nih.gov/16372177/

'... cryotherapy is no more effective than a placebo intervention ... following
a marathon'
https://pubmed.ncbi.nlm.nih.gov/29127510/

'... immerse as much of your body as you can and stay there for 10 minutes'
'The cold truth: the role of cryotherapy in the treatment of injury and
recovery from exercise', PubMed (nih.gov)

'... you now have some justification to opt for a warm shower instead' www
.ncbi.nlm.nih.gov/pmc/articles/PMC6205067/

'... endurance athletes who got less than seven hours a night were more
likely to succumb to injury over the course of a year'
'General health complaints and sleep associated with new injury within an
endurance sporting population: A prospective study', *Journal of Science and
Medicine in Sport* (jsams.org)

'... not getting enough shut-eye has many negative consequences for
running' 'Sleep Hygiene for Optimizing Recovery in Athletes: Review and
Recommendations' (nih.gov)

'... additional sleep (in the form of a nap) only influenced time to exhaustion in runners who were already sleep-deprived'
'The influence of an afternoon nap on the endurance performance of trained runners', PubMed (nih.gov)

'... donning a pair of knee-high compression socks for 48 hours after a marathon had a positive effect on recovery'

'Compression Socks and Functional Recovery Following Marathon, *The Journal of Strength and Conditioning Research* (lww.com)

'... tight-wearing cyclists also performed better in a subsequent "all-out" cycling test'
https://pubmed.ncbi.nlm.nih.gov/33835198/

'... could not find any reduction in DOMS when compression socks were worn during – and for six hours after – exercise'
'Multi-Parametric Analysis of Below-Knee Compression Garments on Delayed-Onset Muscle Soreness', PubMed (nih.gov)

'... there was some evidence that it could slightly reduce DOMS and improve post-run flexibility'
'Effect of sports massage on performance and recovery: a systematic review and meta-analysis', *BMJ Open Sport & Exercise Medicine*

# Chapter 10

'... elite male distance runners used 6 per cent less oxygen at a fixed pace than did recreational runners'
'Running economy of elite and non-elite runners' (researchgate.net)

'... smiling improves running economy and lowers rate of perceived exertion, while frowning does the opposite'
'The effects of facial expression and relaxation cues on movement economy, physiological, and perceptual responses during running', ScienceDirect

'... increasing cadence by 10 per cent reduced average peak impact force by 5.6 per cent'
'Effect of Increasing Running Cadence on Peak Impact Force in an Outdoor Environment', PubMed (nih.gov)

'... increasing cadence by 7.5 per cent reduced forces on the knee joint'
'The effects of body-borne loads and cadence manipulation on patellofemoral and tibiofemoral joint kinetics during running', PubMed (nih.gov)

'This finding is often attributed to a study'
'Impact Loading and Locomotor-Respiratory Co-ordination Significantly Influence Breathing Dynamics in Running Humans', (plos.org)

## Chapter 11

'... boosted running economy by 2–8 per cent and time trial or race performance in endurance events by 2–4 per cent'
'How Strength Training Makes You Faster', Outside Online

## Chapter 12

'... what you eat in the two hours following any very hard or very long run, when your immune system will be most severely suppressed'
'Recovery of the immune system after exercise', *Journal of Applied Physiology*

'...14 per cent of runners had suffered chafing within the last year' https://pubmed.ncbi.nlm.nih.gov/33092325/

'... an oral rehydration solution (containing electrolytes) decreased muscle cramp susceptibility in runners, while water did not' https://pubmed.ncbi.nlm.nih.gov/33722257/

'Twelve per cent said they'd got caught short, experiencing faecal incontinence during a run'
https://pubmed.ncbi.nlm.nih.gov/1556421/

'The incidence and severity of symptoms is significantly higher when exercising in hot conditions'
https://pubmed.ncbi.nlm.nih.gov/29234915/

'... also mitigated the effects of the heat on their performance' https://pubmed.ncbi.nlm.nih.gov/24150782/

## Chapter 13

'... strengthening the hip muscles reduced the risk of IT band problems'
'Hip abductor strength and lower extremity running related injury in distance runners: A systematic review', PubMed (nih.gov)

'... research suggests that while most runners believe it to be an important factor, health care professionals rate it less so'
'What are the perceptions of runners and healthcare professionals on footwear and running injury risk?' (nih.gov)

'... no difference in injury risk between using a shoe with a high heel-toe drop or a low heel-toe drop'
'Influence of the Heel-to-Toe Drop of Standard Cushioned Running Shoes on Injury Risk in Leisure-Time Runners: A Randomized Controlled Trial With 6-Month Follow-up', PubMed (nih.gov)

'... found that runners with "pronated" feet experienced fewer injuries when wearing a motion control shoe'

'Injury risk in runners using standard or motion control shoes: a randomised controlled trial with participant and assessor blinding', PubMed (nih.gov)

'... found no association between a pronated foot type and injury rate over the course of a year'
'Foot pronation is not associated with increased injury risk in novice runners wearing a neutral shoe: a 1-year prospective cohort study', PubMed (nih.gov)

'... rotating two or more pairs of shoes was associated with fewer injuries among runners'
'Can parallel use of different running shoes decrease running-related injury risk?', PubMed (nih.gov)

'... inadequate calorie intake to a raised risk of injury, with a particularly strong association to stress fractures' https://journals.humankinetics.com/view/journals/ijsnem/29/2/article-p189.xml

'Similar research in 2017 looked at runners with knee pain' www.ncbi.nlm.nih.gov/pubmed/28476901

'... icing for 10 minutes was just as effective as longer periods in reducing swelling and pain'
'Comparing the antiswelling and analgesic effects of three different ice pack therapy durations: a randomized controlled trial on cases with soft tissue injuries', PubMed (nih.gov)

'... more than 70 per cent using NSAIDS for injuries'
'Amateur endurance athletes' use of non-steroidal anti-inflammatory drugs: a cross-sectional survey', PubMed (nih.gov)

'... there's likely not much to be gained from supplementation if you are not deficient in these particular nutrients' https://journals.humankinetics.com/view/journals/ijsnem/29/2/article-p189.xml

'... potential problems associated with relying on a scan to tell you why you're hurting'
www.nejm.org/doi/full/10.1056/NEJM199407143310201

'... it did reduce pain levels in runners suffering from patellofemoral pain' https://pubmed.ncbi.nlm.nih.gov/29758508/

'... even if it's just a psychological sticking plaster' https://pubmed.ncbi.nlm.nih.gov/30526288/

# Chapter 15

'... the taper enables important physiological adaptations to take place, microcellular damage to heal and accumulated fatigue to ease'
'Tapering, Performance, Endurance Runners' (researchgate.net)

'... A taper's effect on this important performance parameter is most prevalent among less experienced runners'
https://pubmed.ncbi.nlm.nih.gov/15487904/

'... the taper helps reverse this, reducing the risk of infections'
'The effect of tapering period on plasma pro-inflammatory cytokine levels and performance in elite male cyclists', PubMed (nih.gov)

'... increases the rate at which energy can be produced aerobically'
'Physiological changes associated with the pre-event taper in athletes', PubMed (nih.gov)

'... increased power output, as a result of better fast-twitch muscle fibre function'
'Single Muscle Fiber Gene Expression with Run Taper' (nih.gov)

'... a 2015 study from Loughborough University'
'Tapering strategies in elite British endurance runners', PubMed (nih.gov)

'... every single one ran a positive split'
'Age Differences in Pacing in Endurance Running: Comparison between Marathon and Half-Marathon Men and Women' (nih.gov)

'... research suggests that men slow more significantly in the marathon than women'
'Men are more likely than women to slow in the marathon', PubMed (nih.gov)

'... research does support the use of a simple 24-hour carb load as a way of topping up those glycogen stores' www.ncbi.nlm.nih.gov/pmc/articles/PMC6628334/

# Chapter 16

'... people who expected to hit the wall were more likely to!'
'Hitting the wall in the marathon: Phenomenological characteristics and associations with expectancy, gender, and running history', ScienceDirect

'... aids venous return as well as easing swelling and muscle pain'

'hydrostatic pressure: its benefits for aquatic rehabilitation and exercise' (swimex.com)

'Research in the journal *Nutrients*'
'Achieving Optimal Post-Exercise Muscle Protein Remodeling in Physically Active Adults through Whole Food Consumption', *Nutrients* (mdpi.com)

# Chapter 17

'... less than half consumed sufficient carbohydrate, based on sports nutrition recommendations, while 87 per cent met protein guidelines'

'Many non-elite multisport endurance athletes do not meet sports nutrition recommendations for carbohydrates', PubMed (nih.gov)

'... consuming a low-carbohydrate diet (30 per cent) led to higher markers of immune stress during three days of intense training compared to a high-carbohydrate diet (60 per cent)'
'Influence of dietary carbohydrate intake on the free testosterone: cortisol ratio responses to short-term intensive exercise training', PubMed (nih.gov)

'... ideal recovery prescription'
https://pubmed.ncbi.nlm.nih.gov/27789774/

'... researchers found that there were no differences in terms of glycogen replenishment and protein synthesis between them'
'Small portions of fast food just as effective for recovery after work-out as sports supplements', ScienceDaily

'Fat oxidation can increase by as much as 25 per cent through endurance training'
'The Effect of a 3-Month Low-Intensity Endurance Training Program on Fat Oxidation and Acetyl-CoA Carboxylase-2 Expression', *Diabetes* (diabetesjournals.org)

'One study review reported improvement gains ranging from 1–13 per cent in workouts lasting 70 minutes to four hours'
1475-2891-12-16.pdf (biomedcentral.com)

'Despite not actually swallowing the sugary liquid, they still gained performance benefits'
https://pubmed.ncbi.nlm.nih.gov/21660838/

'... a LCHF diet found that despite greater fat oxidation, their economy went down and they experienced a performance *decline*'
'Low carbohydrate, high fat diet impairs exercise economy and negates the performance benefit from intensified training in elite race walkers', PubMed (nih.gov)

'Higher intakes – 70–90g (2½–3oz) carbohydrate per hour – are sometimes recommended for exercise lasting more than two-and-a-half hours' https://pubmed.ncbi.nlm.nih.gov/21660838/

'... such as someone running under three hours for the marathon' https://pubmed.ncbi.nlm.nih.gov/23846824/

'... took in on average just under 15g (½oz) per hour'
'Analysis of nutritional intake in trail runners during competition', PubMed (nih.gov)

## Chapter 18

'Research from Korea'
'Long Distance Runners Present Upregulated Sweating Responses than Sedentary Counterparts' (plos.org)

'In fact, the ad libitum exercisers performed a bit better'
'Impact of Ad Libitum Versus Programmed Drinking on Endurance Performance: A Systematic Review with Meta-Analysis', PubMed (nih.gov)

'... decreased endurance exercise performance by 2.4 per cent compared to a well-hydrated state'
'Impact of Pre-exercise Hypohydration on Aerobic Exercise Performance, Peak Oxygen Consumption and Oxygen Consumption at Lactate Threshold: A Systematic Review with Meta-analysis', PubMed (nih.gov)

'You may also get muscle cramps or headaches, or feel dizzy and confused'
https://pubmed.ncbi.nlm.nih.gov/32825404/

# Chapter 19

'... works its magic most reliably and consistently in aerobic endurance exercise'
'International society of sports nutrition position stand: caffeine and exercise performance', PubMed (nih.gov)

'... rather than just a single pre-exercise dose' https://pubmed.ncbi.nlm.nih.gov/27426699/

'... the benefits endure even in regular caffeine users' https://pubmed.ncbi.nlm.nih.gov/28495846/

'... regardless of whether people abstained from caffeine for four days beforehand or not'
https://pubmed.ncbi.nlm.nih.gov/21279864/

'... the effects of beetroot on exercise performance in October 2020'
'Ergogenic Effect of Nitrate Supplementation: A Systematic Review and Meta-analysis' (nih.gov)

'... there was a clear, though small, ergogenic effect'
www.ncbi.nlm.nih.gov/pmc/articles/PMC5295087/

'... the magnitude of performance improvement has not been found to differ between recreational and elite athletes' www.liebertpub.com/doi/10.1089/jcr.2011.0022

'... which helps protect against bone mineral loss'
www.ncbi.nlm.nih.gov/pmc/articles/PMC6721335/

'... with readings between 30 and 49nmol/L considered "inadequate"'
'Vitamin D' (nih.gov)
www.ncbi.nlm.nih.gov/pmc/articles/PMC6721335/
'... in Australia, anything below 50nmol/L is considered deficient'

'Vitamin D in athletes: focus on physical performance and musculoskeletal injuries', PubMed (nih.gov)

'... if your level is below 50nmol/L, you would be advised to up your daily dose'
'Distribution of vitamin D status in the UK: a cross-sectional analysis of UK Biobank', *BMJ Open*

# RESOURCES

## Race prediction tools

omnicalculator.com
Click on Sports, and you'll find a range of running calculators, from a race predictor to a 'percent improvement' calculator (i.e. if you improved by 1 per cent, your performance would change from X to Y) and a marathon pace calculator.

mcmillanrunning.com
US coach Greg McMillan's website offers race predictions for and from anything from 100m (110 yards) to 100 miles (160km) as well as giving comprehensive training pace guidelines associated with your specific goal and current fitness.

runnersworld.com
This offers a range of race and pace prediction tools, including a print-your-own pace band.

## Route planning apps

strava.com
The biggest training app out there – use it to log and review your runs, create new routes, check out other runners' activities and download them to try yourself. Free to use, but paid subscription offers extra data and features, such as personalised route suggestions.

plotaroute.com
My preferred tool for route planning, though it doesn't double up as a training tool or log. You can put in two places and ask it to plot you a route, or build a route by hand, using your chosen trails or roads, getting distance and elevation information as you go.

mapmyrun.com
Create and discover routes in your area, save your favourites and find popular routes in any major city when you're travelling. You can plot a route retrospectively to see how far it was and get other route data.

komoot.com
Great for trail runners, Komoot offers ready-built routes in your area that can be filtered by distance, difficulty or even public transport links. It provides details about the terrain, too.

gojauntly.com
Designed primarily for walking, this app lets you pick the greenest, quietest, less-polluted route between A and B as well as suggesting circular routes from your doorstep.

## Finding a running club or group

englandathletics.org (governing body for England)
Go to Clubs and Facilities and you'll find a search tool to locate affiliated running clubs or 'Run Together' groups in your area by postcode or town.

runtogether.co.uk
This is the 'recreational' arm of England Athletics and its website will enable you to find your nearest registered 'Run Together' groups.

scottishathletics.org.uk (governing body for Scotland)
Go to Club Finder and search by location or affiliated club name – filter by discipline, if you like – e.g. hill running, ultrarunning, road running...

jogscotland.org.uk
Find one of nearly 300 free Jog Scotland groups. Despite the name, Jog Scotland groups are not only for beginners. They have intermediate and advanced groups, too.

welshathletics.org (governing body for Wales)
Go to Find a Club to locate an affiliated running club in Wales.

irun.wales
Rhedeg Cymru (Run Wales) is the 'social' running option, offering mostly free running groups across the nation to inspire, encourage and support runners.

athleticsni.org (governing body for Northern Ireland)
Northern Ireland's governing body for running has over 90 affiliated clubs.

joggingbuddy.com
Find someone to run with, wherever you are, by registering with Jogging Buddy.

## Finding a coach

Running coaches should hold a licence issued by their nation's governing body (the organisations outlined above). The best way to find one is through recommendation, but you could also try the following companies, which have coaches/locations across the country:

runningschool.com

we-run.co.uk

whichtrainingcamp.com (go to Find a Coach)

If you're looking specifically for running form coaching, try run3d.co.uk, who have affiliated clinics throughout the UK and Europe.

## Lesser-known kit and shoe brands to check out

altrarunning.eu/uk
All models are zero drop.

alpkit.com
UK-based apparel, accessories and head torches.

inov-8.com
Specialists in trail running.

sundried.com
Good sustainability credentials.

lululemon.co.uk
High-quality Canadian running apparel.

tekoforlife.co.uk
Eco-friendly merino wool running socks.

tracksmith.com/gb
Beautifully designed but pricey apparel.

provizsports.com
High-viz clothing and accessories.

boobydoo.co.uk
Sports bra specialists with a wide range of brands.

## Rucksacks, hydration packs and accessories

ospreyeurope.com
Bags of all shapes and sizes.

camelbak.co.uk
Specialists in hydration packs.

inov-8.com
Race vests.

salomon.com
Race vests and rucksacks.

ultimatedirection.com
Running backpacks, vests, belts and fuel accessories.

nathansports.com
Fuel belts, bags, accessories, lights and high viz.

flipbelt.co.uk
Running belts.

spibelt.com
Running belts.

petzl.com
Running head torches.

## Compression gear brands

cepsports.co.uk

compressport.com

skinscompression.com

uk.2xu.com

## Finding a sports medicine therapist

csp.org.uk
Chartered Society of Physiotherapy. Click on 'Find a physio' to find a qualified chartered physiotherapist in your area.

thesma.org
The Association for Soft Tissue Therapists. 'Find a practitioner' will list registered and qualified sports massage and other manual therapists across the country.

osteopathy.org.uk
The General Osteopathic Council. Find a registered osteopath using the postcode or town search feature.

## Running cadence tools

getcadence.app
This is a free app that will tell you what your cadence is, if you don't have a device that does.

metronome.app
To improve cadence, download Metronome Beats, with which you can set a tempo and rhythm.

## Strength training equipment

physicalcompany.co.uk

This is an Aladdin's cave of fitness equipment, from resistance bands and loops to hand weights, kettlebells, barbells, exercise mats and steps.

TK Maxx and Decathlon are also good bets.

## Running health

2Toms SportShield (they also do a BlisterShield) is my tried-and-trusted choice of anti-chafe product – available as a roll-on or powder.

Leaping Fish Original Runners Rub is a good natural (vegan) option.

Brands worth checking out for physio tape include Kinesio, KT tape and RockTape.

## Finding a race

These websites allow you to search for events by location, date and distance. Some include reviews so you can see how other runners have rated them:

letsdothis.com

findarace.com

runbritain.com (UK only)

racecheck.com

## Race tour and travel companies

whichtrainingcamp.com

sportstoursinternational.co.uk

209events.com

## Finding a sports nutritionist

bda.uk.com
This is the Association of UK Dietitians – they hold the Sport and Exercise Nutrition Register of qualified and experienced practitioners working with athletes of all levels.

precisionhydration.com
This site specialises in hydration advice and services, including sweat testing.

www.performancefood.co.uk
A sports nutrition consultancy run by Dr Karen Reid, a Registered Dietician and Sport & Exercise Nutritionist who has worked at an elite level in high performance sport over the past 25 years.

# APPENDIX 1

## CARB AND PROTEIN CONTENT IN COMMON FOODS

### How much carbohydrate in...?

*(Figures are in grams per portion stated, rounded up or down to nearest whole figure.)*

| | |
|---|---:|
| 1 medium banana | 35g |
| 1 apple | 20g |
| 1 orange | 15g |
| 1 x 80g serving grapes (10–15 grapes) | 12g |
| 6 dried apricots | 25g |
| 1 carton natural yoghurt (150g) | 34g |
| 1 teaspoon honey | 12g |
| 1 heaped teaspoon (15g) strawberry jam | 9g |
| 1 slice wholemeal bread (40g) | 15g |
| 1 wholemeal pitta bread | 27g |
| 3 oatcakes | 18g |
| 1 average bagel (10cm/4in diameter) | 39g |
| 1 potato farl | 21g |
| 1 slice malt loaf | 22g |
| 50g muesli | 35g |
| 2 Weetabix | 25g |
| 50g (medium) serving All-Bran | 24g |
| 45g serving porridge oats | 26g |

| | |
|---|---|
| 500ml (17fl oz) semi-skimmed milk | 25g |
| 1 cereal bar (30g) | 19g |
| 1 bottle sports drink | 30g |
| 1 large jacket potato | 80g |
| 1 medium sweet potato (250g) | 51g |
| 1 serving (75g uncooked weight) brown basmati rice | 54g |
| 1 small tin baked beans (207g) | 45g |
| 1 serving hummus (50g) | 6g |
| 1 serving cottage cheese (100g) | 4g |
| 1 wholewheat tortilla | 16g |
| 1 serving (85g uncooked weight) spaghetti | 63g |

## How much protein in...?

*(Figures are in grams per portion stated, rounded up or down to nearest whole figure.)*

| | |
|---|---|
| 1 carton (150g) natural yoghurt | 8g |
| 500ml semi-skimmed milk | 18g |
| 50g muesli | 5g |
| 1 average bagel (10cm/4in diameter) | 8g |
| 50g (medium) serving All-Bran | 7g |
| 1 large egg | 7g |
| 25g (a palmful) mixed seeds | 7g |
| 25g (a palmful) almonds | 6g |
| 1 heaped teaspoon (15g) peanut butter | 4g |
| 80g tinned tuna in brine | 14g |
| 1 chicken breast (125g) | 30g |
| 1 salmon fillet (150g) | 30g |
| 1 small lean fillet steak (115g) | 28g |
| 1 standard tin sardines in brine (120g) | 20g |
| 3 oatcakes | 3g |
| 1 x 40g piece (matchbox size) Cheddar cheese, grated | 10g |
| 1 serving cottage cheese (100g) | 11g |
| 1 buffalo mozzarella ball (125g) | 21g |
| 1 x 50g serving feta cheese | 8g |
| ½ standard tin of kidney beans | 9g |
| 1 pack prepared Puy lentils | 10g |
| 1 small tin (207g) baked beans | 10g |

| | |
|---|---:|
| 1 serving tofu (100g) | 12g |
| 1 serving hummus (50g) | 3g |
| 1 wholemeal pitta bread | 6g |
| 1 slice wholemeal bread | 4g |
| 1 orange | 1.5g |
| 1 peach or nectarine | 1.5g |

# APPENDIX 2

# MONITORING INTENSITY TABLE

| Level | Type of run | How does it feel? | Talk Test | |
|-------|-------------|-------------------|-----------|---|
| 1 | Easy runs, easy long runs | Like you could continue indefinitely without much effort | Easy to chat | |
| 2 | Steady runs, some long runs or sections of long runs | A moderate effort that makes you breathe a bit harder | Still conversational, albeit more breathlessly than level 1 | |
| 3 | Tempo and lactate threshold runs | On the edge of your comfort zone. Controlled discomfort/comfortably hard. Breathing is fast but rhythmic and controlled | Only short phrases of conversation are possible | |
| 4 | VO$_2$ max efforts | Tough. Challenging. Breathing may be ragged | One-word answers only! | |
| 5 | Sprints | Like you're going as hard as you can. The duration of the efforts is short, however, so your breathing won't be challenged (until after it's finished!) | None. Some sprinters even hold their breath | |

| RPE (on Borg 1–10 scale) | Pace | Heart Rate (as percentage of maximum) | Notes |
|---|---|---|---|
| 1–2 (really easy to somewhat easy) | A guideline might be 90–105 secs slower than goal marathon pace, but less-fast runners may find this results in too slow a pace | 60–70% of MHR | Runs described as 'easy' or 'very easy' fit here |
| 3–4 (moderate to somewhat hard) | A guideline might be 30 secs slower than goal marathon pace, but again this tends to work better for quicker runners. For others, steady pace may be equal to marathon pace or a little faster, up to half-marathon pace | 70–79% of MHR | Efforts described as steady, or at marathon pace and up to half-marathon pace, could fit this category |
| 5–7 (hard to very hard) | Likely to tally with the pace you could sustain in a race for one hour | Around 85%-90% of MHR (closer to 90% for quicker runners) | Efforts run at '10K pace/effort' will generally fit these guidelines |
| 8–9 (Very very hard) | Likely to be run at paces between your 1-mile and 5K race pace | 92–100% of MHR | Efforts run at 1 mile, 3K and 5K pace/effort will generally fit these guidelines |
| 10 (maximal) | All-out! | Not relevant as not aerobic, and because it cannot be measured quickly enough | Hill sprints and flat sprints |

# ACKNOWLEDGEMENTS

I'm really grateful to Charlotte Croft and all the team at Bloomsbury for making this book happen.

With heartfelt thanks to physiotherapist Mark Buckingham (wpbphysio.co.uk), not just for keeping me on the road but for his great input to the Be a Stronger Runner chapter. Also my thanks to Dr Karen Reid (performancefood.co.uk) for her useful feedback on the Nutrition and Hydration section and to physio Tom Goom (running-physio.com) for letting me share his Ready to Run checklist in Chapter 13.

Most of all, though, I want to thank Jeff Pyrah, my husband and fellow runner, for our almost continuous conversation about running over the last decade and a half!

# INDEX